Reasons or Results!

Be Your Own Personal Trainer

How To Get
Exceptional Fitness Results,

During Your
First Three-months,

And Build A Foundation
For Lifelong Success.

**Free 1-hour consultation
with the author with purchase of this book.**

by

Sov Valentine,
Fat-loss Specialist
CFT, Cft, SPN, SSC, GFI, YFI, SFI, CMCht, Reiki Master, CERT, LFR

20+ years professional experience.

https://sovereign-valentine.mykajabi.com

About The Author

Sovereign Valentine has invested the last four decades studying, experimenting and applying general fitness principles, as well as perfecting the fat-loss principles contained herein. He has 37 years experimenting and applying nutrition and close to 30 years as a personal trainer and health professional.

After witnessing first-hand, the affects of poor lifestyle choices within his family and breaking free of the junk food and sugar addiction behaviors himself, he has been refining and practicing what he preaches for the last three decades. During that time, Sov personally invested tens-of-thousands of dollars experimenting to find out what products and ideas are hoaxes and which ones are actually effective and work with those who commit to applying them.

Through an intensive and extensive trial-and-error process and by consistently doing what was purported to work he found what really *does* work. He then goes about documenting the results with each client.

In Sov's words, *"There is no longer a mystery to healthy, sustainable fat-loss. The science and art have been figured out...there aren't any exceptions...it simply comes down to doing the correct things at the correct times and refining as you go. If you think you're an exception, you're not!"*

Sovereign began his formal training as a health care professional with a sincere desire to work with athletes. From a combination of formal training and experimenting, he developed a system that absolutely works.

Sovereign says, *"If you aren't burning between 12 to 20 pounds of fat per month, something is off. A properly designed and executed exercise and nutrition program will facilitate these numbers, (as well as improve overall health) unless you aren't following-through correctly. Without a way to know if you're on track, weeks could go by and you wouldn't even know if you're off track."*

In 1992, he became a Licensed Massage Therapist in Washington State. In 1994 he began doing small, informal nutrition presentations so that others could experience the profound impact that real nutrition has on the body. In 1996, he became a foot and hand reflexologist as well as an energetic healing master. In 1997, he became a certified hypno-therapist. In 1998, he began training others in hypnotherapy and in 1999 he became the first person ever at The Gabriel Institute to be certified as a Master Clinical Hypnotherapist. He went on to become certified in Fitness Training, Fitness Therapy, Sports Conditioning, Endurance Conditioning, a Specialist in Performance Nutrition as well as a Youth Conditioning Specialist, Golf Fitness Instructor, Senior Fitness Specialist and Community Emergency Response Team Member and Licensed Emergency First Responder.

Sovereign's thorough understanding of the systems of the body and how they relate to one another is reflected in his ability to fine-tune his client's training and nutritional regimes for extra-ordinary *Results!* His published works include:

- *Reasons or Results Performance Nutrition Training.*

- *Weighting To Wait; The Emotions of Permanent Fat-loss.*

- *Be Your Own Personal Trainer.*

- *If I were her Trainer.*

- *50-ish Reasons: Why actively and purposely withholding the B.N.B.B.s from your boy is a really bad idea*

Foreword

The fitness, nutrition and weight loss industries have been evolving over the last hundred-years, but especially so in the last forty-years, as being overweight and obese, as well as diabetes and all the other *dis*-eases that accompany being overweight have increased to epidemic proportions.

Generally speaking, the amount of available health and fitness information is simply crazy. But accurate, science-based information which produces healthy, consistent results that can be maintained over the long haul is simple in nature, but challenging to isolate. Much of what's out there is simply about spewing marketing and advertising solutions for some problem symptoms (being overweight and in pain) and then saying, *"Here, take this and all your problems will be solved."*

The truth of the matter, after applying this kind of information for more than three decades, on both myself and with my clients, is that there truly are good nutritional products that make weight loss easier, faster and with less effort, but they are few and far between and the general public simply can't tell a good product from an ineffective one. That's a part of what I do...*assure quality and success through health improvement to prevent and reduce suffering.*

In the United States right now, the right people are doing the right research to help you get real *Results!* At the same time, most food products and dietary supplements for sale really have little nutrition at all, resulting in a lot of missed opportunities by people who could have gotten better *Results!* but to this day don't know why they don't know.

When you hear the words 'fad diet', what they're talking about is either a good program that people picked away at until there wasn't any relevant nutritional content left (requires lifestyle change). Or, the program promised weight loss, fitness and athletic results without exercise and nutritional-density to begin with. With any health and fitness program, if the amount of nutritional-density isn't increased and isn't provided to your body consistently, you simply won't stick with it since there's no pay off to your chemistry of the brain and body, without additional, consistent nutrition-density.

Secondly, any program that suggests you can burn off all the fat and gain health in all ways, but is without some kind of resistance-training [and] cardiovascular/aerobic exercise, its a pipe dream designed to appeal to people who feel frustrated, depressed, sad, defeated and helpless...feeling like they can't do it anymore...empty promises...*hype*...- a bait-and-switch.

The true secret is finding a trainer who has your overall health in mind (not just short-term results) [your health should be improving and you should be feeling better as time goes on] and a trainer who has enough expertise to not only design an amazingly effective program, but one who knows how to adjust the program to you for most effectiveness. Most trainers can design a program, but many don't know how to adjust the program if progress slows down or progress hits a plateau (accountability for both the client and the trainer). This is the second part of what I do.

One of the things that makes me so effective as a trainer is that I've been doing this so long, that when a client isn't getting results, I can narrow it down to whether it has something with the actual workouts, the thoughts & attitudes of the client, the nutritional aspect or if it's in the application of the program during the hours when the client isn't with me.

There simply aren't any mysteries to healthy, sustainable fat-loss to me anymore. A majority of trainers don't stick with the industry long enough to find out what *they didn't know*...I have.

This book lays it out there in simple, concise form and states the basics from many angles and view points, so there's no question what has to happen as you progress through this book.

When you apply these tactics in the way I show you here, you and those who know you will be blown away by the *Results!* you are getting. This book is for people who want the results that speak for themselves...anyone can get some results in the short-run...every 'die-it' will produce some kind of results in the short-run, but most quick, fitness programs erode the physical health after leaving you malnourished, tired, exhausted and depleted...resulting in decreased health and vitality.

Any health-building fitness program should leave you feeling lighter, clearer, relaxed, rejuvenated and more vital than when you started, as well as free of all cravings and any attraction to junk food.

Apply this information and you will be so glad you did…*I promise.*

Read this book now; start getting better today and I look forward to seeing and hearing how good you feel about the *Results!* you are getting!

Once you've read the material, if you're the type to recognize what is real and not just the next fad and if you're willing to commit and follow through until the end, *I'll be there with you every step of the way.*

Acknowledgments

I have not attempted to cite in the text all the authorities and sources in the preparation of this book. To do so would require more space than is available, in order to effectively serve you who apply this information. The list would include departments of the federal government, libraries, industrial institutions, web sources and many individuals as well as my personal experiences and those of my clients since the late 1980's.

Inspiration was contributed by all those before me who succeeded as best they could with the information they had at the time, as well as all those after me who will improve upon this information to make the lives of others better. This book is a culmination of hundreds of books I read, thousands of hours of experimentation and thousands of hours of observing the why, how and where of my own and others' successes and failures.

A Word From The Author

Do it!

This is a *do it* book…read it, learn it…*do it.* If you don't apply it as instructed you'll miss out. Reading this book provides the information but is not the same as doing.

If you need help, contact me!

I work to make a living, but I live to see you get *Results!*

Sovereign Michael Valentine,

April 2018.

Disclaimer

This book is designed to provide information about the subject matter covered. It is produced and sold with the understanding that the publisher and author are not engaged in rendering neither medical diagnosis nor treatment. If you need medical help, go get it. It is not the purpose of this manual to reprint all the information that is otherwise available from other health professionals, but to complement, amplify and supplement other texts. *Reasons or Results! Life-long Fat-loss Program* is neither a cure-all nor a quick-fix for poor lifestyle habits or tendencies. Anyone who commits to personal accountability for their health must expect to re-direct some time, energy and money without any guarantee for specific benefits within a fixed time frame. *Nature works at her own pace.*

Every effort has been made to make this book as complete and accurate as possible. However, there may be mistakes both typographical and in content. Therefore, this book should be used as a general guide and not as the ultimate source of health and nutritional information. Your uniqueness will shine through as you succeed.

The purpose of this book is to educate and inform. The very best results will come from participation. Neither the publisher nor the author shall have responsibility to any person or entity with respect to any loss or damage caused by or alleged to be caused directly or indirectly by the information contained in this book.

This book is not meant to replace the advice or treatments prescribed by your doctor, but rather to accompany your physician's advice. It is not meant to encourage medical treatment of illness or disease or any medical problem by the layperson. It is meant to inform you and open you to health choices that are available to those who seek a broader knowledge. Any application of the ideas set forth in this book is at the applicant's discretion and sole risk. If you are under a doctor's care for any condition, she or he can advise you *about information she or he is familiar with and which she or he has personally experienced.*

The information in this book is neither diagnostic nor prescriptive. It is informational only. The data and information contained herein are based upon information from various peer-reviewed, published and unpublished sources and merely represent training, experience, health and nutrition literature and practices summarized.

Neither the publisher nor the author of this book makes any warranties, expressed or implied regarding the currency, completeness or scientific accuracy or validity of this information nor does it warrant the fitness of the information for any particular purpose. It is intended to provide helpful and informative material on the subjects addressed in the publication. It is sold with the understanding that the publisher and author are not engaged in rendering medical, health, or any other kind of personal professional services in this book. The publisher and author specifically disclaim all responsibility for any liability, loss or risk, personal or otherwise which is incurred as a consequence, directly or indirectly, from the use and application of any of the contents of this book.

Table of Contents

About The Author   5

Foreword   7

Acknowledgements   10

A Word From The Author   11

Disclaimer   12

Definitions   16

Introductions   20

Chapter One: What You Get   27

Chapter Two: What Exactly Do I Mean?   33

Chapter Three: Off-setting Genetic Potential   39

Chapter Four: Structure And Definitions   43

Chapter Five: The Next 90 Days   54

Chapter Six: Defining Your Goals   67

Chapter Seven: The Four Key Questions   76

Chapter Eight: Resistance-Training   82

Chapter Nine: Fat-Burning Cardio   90

Chapter Ten: How To Measure Body Composition   101

Chapter Eleven: What The Numbers Mean   104

Chapter Twelve: What The Body Comp Percentages Mean   118

Chapter Thirteen: Rob Rector's Success   122

Chapter Fourteen: Basics Of Advanced, Applied Nutrition   139

Chapter Fifteen: Functional-Foods   152

Chapter Sixteen: Whole-foods   159

Chapter Seventeen: Recovery   176

Chapter Eighteen: Common Sticking Points   182

Chapter Nineteen: Motivation   197

Pre-training Questionnaire   211

Afterword   213

Appendix   215

Definitions

1) B.N.B.B.s: Basic Nutritional Building Blocks; concentrated food in tablet, capsule and powder form, including:

Functional-foods designed to elicit a certain physiological response at certain times: *e.g. stabilize blood sugar level, recovery post-workout, replace electrolytes.*

Generally speaking, functional–foods are foods which have a higher level of nutrition than non, functional-foods, but more convenient and economical, in nature

The B.N.B.B.s:

- Some sort of protein,

- Multi-vitamin/mineral,

- Good-fats,

- *Pro*-biotics,

- Vitamin B-Complex,

- Vitamin C-Complex,

- Vitamin E-Complex,

- Dietary Fiber and

- Clean drinking water.

2)) *De*-generation: the slow, [often with seemingly sudden onset] process of gradual and preventable breakdown of the essential systems and capabilities of the body.

*When the body doesn't have the B.N.B.B.s and it begins to break down, malfunction, dys-function, manifest syndromes, symptoms, signs, aches, pains, and include fat-gain.

3) *Dis*-ease: the symptoms, mal-functions, dys-functions, syndromes, aches, pains and signs letting us know the process of *de*-generation is well on its way because the cells need the B.N.B.B.s...*dis*-ease(s), are considered normal and average in much of the medical community to those professionals who do not know about the B.N.B.B.s [through first-hand, personal experience].

*Italics added to [*de*-generative] and [*dis*-ease] as a reminder that they are 'processes' which can be interrupted, rather than 'things we have to live with or have no influence over.

4) S.A.D.C.R.A.P. = Standard American Diet of Continuously & Repetitively Advertised Products:

S.A.D.C.R.A.P. includes but is not limited to:

- Soda pop

- Carbonated beverage

- Candy

- Chips

- Ice cream

- Caffeine

- Alcohol

- Tobacco

Anything with partially-hydrogenated oil, artificial fats, artificial sweetener, artificial coloring, artificial preservatives.

5) Complete Recovery Drink: must be a combination of protein & carbohydrate in a ratio of 2.7 (divide protein grams by carbohydrate grams), re-fuel the body following exercise, training, competition as well as recover from injury, illness, *de*-generation & *dis*-ease.

6) "The Black-Forest of chasing symptoms": refers to the process whereby people taking note of or being diagnosed with a particular health problem, symptom, sign, syndrome and/or *de*-generative *dis*-ease and so forth cover up the underlying symptoms with medication...only to have another symptom appear from the medication itself which in-turn gets covered up with another medication…which in-turn gets covered up by another medication…eventually to find their health so *de*-generated and mixed-up that things seem bleak and hopeless.

7) "Search-and-Consume Mode": when someone has waited too long to eat or drink and they reach for whatever will get them some energy the most quickly…often S.A.D.C.R.A.P.…which often leads to a sharp increase in energy followed by a sharp decrease in energy…leading to yet another "search-and-consume-mode"…which cumulatively and ultimately takes one into the black-forest of *de*-generative *dis*-ease.

Every cell of the body [requires] the B.N.B.B.s to maintain, repair and rejuvenate themselves. MOST people are not getting enough B.N.B.B.s for their basic requirements, let alone to burn off excess fat and improve blood chemistry. There are no exceptions. One cannot know if they have enough of them until they do have enough and things that seemed normal simply go away.

Often people attending one of my lectures or reading one of my books will ask, "Yay, but what about my…?" What's the answer?

The B.N.B.B.s!

Yes, some of the cells and systems require other things in addition, but you want to make sure the basics are in place, instead of skipping the basics and substituting other things.

Just like breathing air.

Just like drinking water.

Just like eating food.

Every cell requires them.

One might wonder… *"I have such and such,"* or *"I was diagnosed with this or that…what should I take?"*

Begin with the B.N.B.B.s.

Build upon the B.N.B.B.s.

Every cell requires them.

Done properly, you'll feel so much better and most likely be surprised by all the benefits you experience.

People will be asking you, *"What has changed?…you seem different."*

Introductions

"Until we boldly separate the two concepts of food & nutrition from one another there will always be confusion, debate and resulting subpar nutrition in the body, resulting in subpar body composition (too much fat). The confusion lies in the "one or the other" debate (food or dietary supplements?). Food doesn't necessarily provide consistent enough nutrition and nutrition-density isn't necessarily provided by what we call/think of as food. I've never seen an exception to this." -Sov

For those of us in the fitness industry with enough field experience to *reflect* upon (from the inside out), the relative strengths and weaknesses of the training system we go through and the information provided to us as health professionals for our certification(s), we realize there is a vast ethical, moral and cognitive dissonance between:

What the consumer of weight-loss marketing information wants to believe is intuitive, in terms of what they need to do to lose 'weight' (what we think is right action):

e.g. "Eat less to lose weight."

What the consumer of weight-loss marketing information wants to believe is intuitive, in terms of what they need to do to *burn 'fat'* (what we think is right action):

e.g. "As long as I weigh less and
get smaller, I don't care how it happens."

How much of what is marketed to the consumer of weight-loss marketing information to personal-trainers, fitness trainers and the like pick up and believe to be *credible, safe and effective* in the long-run (for their clients), and in turn apply or get their clients to "do" as ways of attempting to ratify their own value of service, (promise certain *results* to gain a client followed, with no way of holding themselves accountable to potential weight-loss goals let alone health improvements for the clients):

e.g. "As long as the client loses weight and gets smaller they won't know if they have done it safely or not and the trainers don't care as long as they get paid."

What is *quick, convenient,* mediocre in terms of safety, noticeable and yet un-sustainable by the lay-person vs. what is *sustainably fast, safe, easy, noticeable,* as well as clinically measurable as health-promoting, in the short and long-run for improvement of body composition as well as long-term health:

e.g. The main focus is on the client losing weight in the first six-weeks, regardless whether it is safe and healthy or not.

And finally, the fitness professional's ability to discern between what is weight-loss marketing 'hype' (advertising disguised as information or science to keep a consumer wanting to lose weight as long as possible…keep them buying stuff which promises weight loss, *delivers* little and makes the body crave things which cause weight gain):

e.g. Even many personal trainers don't know if the information and direction they are providing is safe for their clients, but they don't know how to measure 'safe' let alone hold themselves accountable to ethical practices."

[And its application should therefore be avoided both by consumers and by fitness professionals due to short-term weight-loss in trade for *long-term health* distortion]:

*e.g. Just because someone loses weight does not mean they got healthier in the process…health should be the first priority, followed by fat-loss…neither are exclusive…*and what is practical, applicable, re-producible science (and its application should not only be adhered to by consumers and health professionals due to short and long-term, sustainable fat-loss but also for clinically measurable and documentable improvements in bio-chemical markers, *e.g. blood pressure, total cholesterol, HDL, LDL, triglyceride levels, blood sugar, insulin sensitivity, etc.* for the top ten *de*-generative *dis*-eases of our time, *e.g. heart dis-ease, diabetes, stroke, obesity, etc.*):

e.g. When one burns fat safely, the chemistry of the body improves, and the overall health improves and can be measured by your physician…if the above markers didn't improve, there may be too much emphasis placed on 'weight-loss' first without regard for health.

Which is the *metabolically and physiologically sound* and yet largely neither marketed nor promoted nor understood by much of the average fitness professional and even less understood by the weight-loss consumer market?

e.g. "I believe relatively few fitness professionals know the difference between weight-loss and fat-loss or the differences in facilitating the two."...for example, a few of the many common and misunderstood concepts regarding weight loss:

- Low fat diets,

- Good vs. bad fat,

- High protein diets,

- Calorie restriction,

- Low carbohydrate diets,

- Attempts at "starving the fat"

- Frequency of meals and snacks,

- Withholding of nutrition-density,

- Quality vs. quantity of fat consumption,

- Exercise without application of nutrition,

- Attempts at weight loss without application of nutrition and

- Attempts at weight loss success, through deprivation and malnutrition.

e.g. The things which don't work in the long-run.

These have been shown to *produce* short-term weight-loss (loss of lean mass along with some body fat), and accompanying disintegration of critical blood-chemistry markers of health *e.g. blood pressure, total cholesterol, HDL, LDL, triglyceride levels, blood sugar, insulin sensitivity, etc.* followed by re-bound *affects* (re-gaining the weight and more):

e.g. The diet market promotes the concept of the quick-fix without regard for the long-term affects...taking advantage of people's desperation while the practical, applicable, *re-producible* science:

• Improves bone mass

• Improves lean mass

• Improves blood pressure, total cholesterol, HDL, LDL, triglyceride levels, blood sugar, insulin sensitivity, etc.) and

• Decreases body fat

e.g. Do it correctly and your whole
life will improve and get better with time.

The themes repeated throughout this book

are done so *purposely* and with great intent,

for the people who need them most,

and are by no stretch of the imagination a coincidence.

It's not uncommon that when the average person *seeks professional training* they are afraid of what they'll be told. They're afraid to be told anything different than what they want to believe or want to believe is true. They're afraid that they'll be told to do things that interfere with the lifestyle they have created which got them to a place the no longer want to be at or that they are no longer satisfied with. *People like to hear their ideas are correct and they are right even when they aren't.* There's a vast difference between being fit, healthy and vital and being right.

People are *so right* today, that 80% of the population is overweight...how can we be fat and out of shape and wrong?

In this way, the greatest challenge for trainers is helping people understand, comprehend and correlate how their thinking has gotten them to a place they want to get away from.

The very best trainers introduce *ideas* in such a way that a person can feel right learning, never noticing that what they are learning might be the opposite of what/how they *wish* things were or how they insist things are even as they get further and further from the best versions of themselves.

You'll likely *get some new ideas*, herein...maybe they sound like old ideas...but the difference is in *applying them to yourself* versus debating, theorizing, hypothesizing and processing, yet never applying. *Getting* super *fit* and healthy *is easy* when you just do *what works* and don't interfere in your own process.

Some points are stated repeatedly throughout this book in every conceivable manner, in response to every question I've heard since I started experimenting with nutrition at age 12...to leave absolutely no question, no matter which angle you perceive the points, what I mean by what I'm saying...*unequivocal clarity.*

These are not just ideas...these are *proven principles* I've been applying with myself for close to thirty-seven years and with my family, friends and clients for twenty-five plus years. The only thing that can get in your way now is what you tell yourself about this information.

Go for it!

Until we boldly separate the two concepts of food & nutrition, from one another, there will always be confusion, debate and resulting subpar nutrition in the body, resulting in subpar health and performance.

The confusion is in, "one or the other" (food or dietary supplements?).

Food doesn't necessarily provide consistent enough nutrition and nutrition-density isn't necessarily provided, by what we call/think of as food.

The result is subpar performance and *bodyfat* that won't seem to *go away or stay away*.

Chapter One

What You Get From
Be Your Own Personal Trainer

Create a new ending, *for the story of your life!*

What I'm going to show you within these pages is how to *get started* on a new level of fitness and health *correctly, safely and effectively,* during any given three-month period. Whether you're completely new and a beginner to health and fitness or you're somewhat experienced and have taken time off or you're very experienced, but simply overwhelmed with all the seeming choices available, in terms of exercises and programs, you can still *expect* to get *amazing results* with this program. Maybe you're highly successful and competitive, but have reached a sticking-point. What you'll get from this is clarity and consistent results, which you'll then (I expect) expand and build on.

The primary focus of this program and the kinds of *benefits you can expect* are:

● *Fat-loss* (not just weight loss, but specifically fat-loss; between 12 and 20 pounds of fat-loss per month), unless you're already at your goal body composition, (as long as you apply the three parts of nutrition).

● *Gain in lean mass* (healthy tissue, more of the good stuff we need for optimal health; between one and three pounds per week),

● Significant *gain in strength,*

● Significant improvement in endurance/stamina (regardless of prior experience),

● Improved synergy between all the different parts of your exercise and nutrition program, *so you get better results* than you've ever gotten before (many people apply exercise and nutrition, [bits and pieces] but the number of people whom have a program, where each part amplifies all the other aspects is rare to say the least, even among the most experienced fitness-buffs and athletes, from beginner to Olympic-level.

How to know if your bits and pieces aren't fitting:

If you feel like you're doing everything right, but you aren't getting what you would *expect* from your program (mediocre results) [can't get lean, aren't recovering from workouts, stuck at a plateau with either strength and/or lean mass, plateau in endurance or speed or having health problems/injuries that either sneak up or don't seem to improve or even simply not feeling as good as you want to].

I'll also cover the specific *behaviors*, *actions* and strategies to help *offset the genetic potentials* we know as hereditary conditions (health conditions people think they have to get/live with because others in their family have had them/have been told, by health professionals we can't avoid them) or even genetic problems that have *already begun* to surface as acute or chronic health problems, e.g. diabetes, heart *dis*-ease, asthma, heart problems and/or problems with systems of the body:

- Skeletal system,

- Immune system,

- Nervous system,

- Digestive system,

- Hormone system,

- Skin, hair & nails,

- Respiratory system,

- Reproductive system,

- Cardiovascular & circulatory system and

- Nervous system (brain and peripheral nerves).

As well as how all the *systems work together* with each other. (each system of the body is supposed to work cooperatively), with all the other systems. When the body is in a 'breaking down' [atrophy/*de*-generative *dis*-ease], rather than a 'building up' [hypertrophy/health], the systems of the body seem to fight against each other and your doctors will likely begin chasing symptom after symptom attempting to (but unwittingly) get ahead of the 'breaking down' process, without knowing why the body is breaking down. Also known as chronic, *de*-generative, *dis*-ease; what I refer to as the "Black-forest of chasing symptoms".

Some of the benefits you'll experience by *consistently* applying the principles herein are:

- Improved sleep,

- Resistance to injury,

- Improved mental clarity,

- Greater emotional stability,

- 50% decrease in colds, flu & bugs,

- Assistance in recovery from injury,

- Improved attention & concentration,

- Relief from chronic health conditions,

- More consistent and increased energy,

- Greater clarity and perspective on your own life,

- Better, more properly responsive immune system,

- A decrease in anxiety and nervousness/sense of peace,

- Dramatic improvement in motivation and consistency and

- Elimination of cravings for unhealthy foods & beverages,

It goes without saying that when your exercise and nutrition program/*habits are dialed-in,* every area of *your life improves.* I have *seen* what some might consider unrelated *miracles,* when people get their fitness program together. Even competitive and professional athletes often have questions about their own body and program, partially because they have followed plans that help a lot of people, but don't seem to address their own particular needs.

Fitness vs competitive athletes:

For the sake of discussion herein, athleticism is what competitive athletes do in order to compete (workouts and nutrition), during the training season and career, but fitness is used to describe what the athlete does outside the competitive realm to address their own personal concerns, as well as improving and maintaining health and wellness outside of competition, as well as part of the *de*-conditioning process post-career (off- season/retirement).

It's very common for competitive athletes to be swept up in 'what to do' on a daily basis, during their career, but once they stop competing, all the resources, guidance and structure go away leaving the post-career athlete, to fend for themselves, which doesn't often go very well. If you take the average lifespan of an NFL player being 55 years, you can consider how people who were once some of the top athletes in the world, *de*-generate/atrophy fairly quickly, post-career.

Part of this phenomena is due to the wear-and-tear, during the career and part is due to lack of *health* maintenance & *preservation* and a focus on post-career fitness. Although there is a *great* range in what and who we consider an athlete and what each athlete subjects their body to during their athletic career, some evidence shows that the average athlete lives 67 years, while people in general live 76 years. Regardless of how much abuse or neglect the body has taken or what hereditary conditions are on the menu, *you can get* the body into the *building-up* of health versus the breaking-down, into *dis*-ease process. It's simply *a choice* of how one invests their time, energy and resources. Many physicians I speak with say that about 90% of visits to the doctor are related to lifestyle: lack of fitness and nutrition.

Because there is so much information available, athletes and non-athletes alike get overwhelmed trying to *decide*/sort what to do and how to prioritize their time and energy, often ending up jumping from one thing to another, but without any clear, consistent, concise, precise and *measurable, trackable or predictable results* (body composition and blood chemistry measurements).

By following this program you'll *develop* a way to know when you're on track and once you're on track, recognize how to compare the results you get from variations in your exercise program, so that you *keep* your 'fitness & health *compass' pointed* to True North.

Often, people have so much variation in their program that they don't *get results* in fat-loss, lean mass, strength nor endurance (all examples of adaptation) and then they subsequently *change parts* of their program, without knowing why they changed it, how to *change it* to get a different outcome or even why you would stay with a program or *make a change* to the program.

This is partly why the really good trainers and coaches are worth their weight in gold...preventing a waste of time or eliminating the 'learning curve' most of the population refers to as, *"I worked out for three-months, but didn't get any results...I've tried everything."*

I'm also going to teach you about the importance of body composition, resting heart rate, target heart rate and caloric requirements.

I'm going to go into very specific instructions with regard to resistance-training, fat-burning/cardiovascular training and how to *nail your fat-burning,* target heart rate zone for the fastest fat-loss possible, without losing all your lean mass (muscle, organs, bone density, etc.), to get the very *best results* you can get for the least amount of time, energy and resources.

If you're the type of person who doesn't want to go through the trial-and-error process and *you* simply *want to be shown what to do* to get the very best results for the least amount of wasted time, energy and resources, this book is for you. If you've *fully decided* to commit the time, energy and resources to get phenomenal results...better result than any of your friends or family are getting, this book is *for you!*

There's never a shortage of people who *want to burn fat,* get lean and so on. In America, there does seem to be a pattern of consumers who insist they want a goal (benefits of exercise and nutrition), but don't follow through on their exercise and nutrition, but still *expect the results* of people who have followed through on their exercise and nutrition. If this describes you, I would refer you to my book *Weighting To Wait*, available on Amazon Kindle which addresses the emotional aspects of yo-yo dieting (consistently starting, but not following through). If you tend to start things but not follow through and *expect results* without doing the real work, this is related to unproductive emotional habits.

Let's talk about what you can get done with the information, in this book.

Chapter Two

What Exactly Do I Mean?

What exactly do I mean by fat-loss, lean mass, gain strength, significantly improve endurance and offset genetic potentials??

Fat-loss:

As *you know* from my other books, articles, blog, classes, etc., I distinguish between weight loss and fat-loss. Weight loss is generally unhealthy (since it doesn't consider overall health markers and tends to lower overall vitality and performance) and fat-loss is considered healthy (since it considers blood chemistry markers, bone density, burning fat specifically, balancing the hormones, strength-to-weight ratio, improving overall vitality and performance).

When I talk weight loss, I'm specifically teaching and coaching you to *focus on health, first* and teaching the body to *utilize fat for energy*, rather than getting visually smaller, but actually losing lean mass and strength, ending up as what is referred to as skinny-fat. Skinny-fat is when people look smaller, they say their clothes fit better, they are generally considered skinny, but have a body composition of 20% or higher (thin, but fat) and quite often their blood chemistry numbers deteriorate.

So, *health has to be the first* consideration in a fat-loss program, so that the program and the *results you get* are sustainable. Without health, cravings for junk food get more intense with time, motivation wanes, consistency is pretty impossible. When scale numbers take priority over health, more than likely you'll start a program and within three-months, after some initial success *you'll start* gaining weight back and likely gain more than you lost. This is a very common, *average experience* among Americans.

The way I teach fat-loss, *12- 20 pounds of fat-loss* per month *until you reach your goal body composition* is conservative and I'll give you my very best secrets in here.

If you are relying on outdated 'diet' information from the 1970's, you'll *hear* people talk about *losing more than two pounds of fat per week* being unhealthy...this is outdated. Before the science of nutrition evolved and the art of exercise program design developed, to where it is now, this is the best they could do. But nowadays, the very best trainers know how to structure exercise and nutrition to *dial-in the fat-burning process*, so *you can burn 12-20 pounds of fat per month, while improving your health.* Potentially, people can burn more, but the *middle of the road* for beginners is easier to fathom for people who haven't been successful in the past.

Back in the 1970's the concept of, *"calories-in, calories-out"* became popular and people starting thinking and promoting that *you can* simply reduce calories to *lose weight.* The idea was roughly that 3,500 calories equals one pound of weight (not fat, but weight). So, people were unwittingly *encouraged* to reduce their calories to lose weight (essentially starving the body) which, after a while, subsequently causes the metabolism to slow down, ultimately causing the body to retain fat and then begin gaining fat back, often more than was originally lost.

It's not uncommon for people, including health care providers and personal trainers to still *promote* these antiquated ideas, today. When people don't have significant training or experience and they don't know what else to say, you'll hear something like, *"Just reduce your calories and you'll lose weight."* It's true the scale may look different, but overall health suffers and I'll go into the reasons for this and solutions of this later...the greatest factor being that as *you* reduce calories, so are *you* reducing nutritional-density/quantity, within the diet, which is required to maintain/sustain *fat-loss.*

In order for any fat-loss program to promote health and the results to be sustainable, your lifestyle habits and *how you see yourself* (self-image) has to improve...otherwise, every time a person achieves some success, they'll likely regress back to the previous version of themselves, which is unnecessary. *Lifestyle and identity have to change.*

Ultimately, *you want* your exercise and nutrition strategies to create measurable improvements...that means improvement in two things: 1) Body composition (decrease in body fat) and 2) Marked improvements in blood chemistry (the results of blood lab panel tests by your doctor). Without these two markers, the program isn't improving your health and any results in 'weight loss' will likely be short lived followed by a rebound affect of gaining more weight back than you started with.

Gain lean mass:

When I talk about gaining lean mass, partly what I'm talking about is *improvements in your physique*. More muscle. But lean mass converts over to improved performance and strength-to-weight ratio as well. Strength-to-weight ratio applies more for athletes to reach optimal performance levels (how strong you are compared to overall weight and body composition).

So, visually, as well as the overall shape of your physique will improve and you can gain two pounds of lean mass per week, assuming the three parts of your nutrition program are dialed-in and applied consistently.

Lean mass relates to improving all the healthy tissues of the body...everything except body fat. So, if *you* think in terms of overall health, we're talking improved bone density, improved health of ligaments, tendons, organs, functions, performance and so on...all the good stuff...how *all the* parts and *systems of the body work cooperatively with each other.* Yes, more muscle feels and looks better to most people. With more muscle comes greater confidence. With greater confidence comes more opportunity. With greater opportunity comes improved lifestyle.

Gain strength:

When I talk about gaining strength, it goes far beyond the physical strength that comes from a properly designed program. *Yes,* just about any weight training (resistance-training) program will improve strength within the first three-months. Beyond that there's more to it.

But more importantly, as a person's *physical strength improves* inside their body, their strength in the outside world improves too. I've seen so many cases over the last twenty years, that once a person sticks with their program and gains strength, other areas of their life get's freed-up and things start improving...things that seem unrelated. Opportunities, jobs, relationships, health, income level and so on, *seemingly out of nowhere.*

These kinds of quality of *life improvements* show up as improved self-esteem, improved sense of self-worth, improved health, improved sports performance, improved independence, as well as injury prevention and recovery.

Significantly improve endurance/stamina:

When I think of all the endurance athletes (running, cycling, swimming, rowing, etc.) I've worked with over the years, the common theme has often been that endurance athletes *don't usually lack in work ethic.* But they do tend to have a pattern of pushing themselves really hard without regard for backing up their body, with a proper nutrition program.

The main themes here are that the training aspects for endurance athletes is mostly in place (although overtraining tends to be a factor). work ethic, pushing themselves, striving, motivation and all that is usually *good to go.* What is generally missing is any *significant understanding* or application of core, applied nutrition strategies (consistent consuming too little/sub-par nutrition-density) and often avoidance of resistance-training.

In other words, most endurance athletes aren't coming close to their potential in performance nor coming close to how *good* they can *feel* in the process. In case you didn't catch that little hint, the *better you feel* on the inside the better your sports performance becomes. There is a direct correlation between how good you feel and how well you perform.

It's not uncommon for runners and cyclists to have all time personal best training sessions, within the first week, of applying the nutrition principles I'll teach *you* in here. Part of the reason for this is that historically, the conditioning aspect has been consistently applied, even beyond fitness to more of a 'toughening' affect (withholding proper sports nutrition, from the body but pushing it to perform anyway).

Once the body begins getting proper, quality nutrition the athlete feels as though the body has been "plugged-in" for the first time. With proper performance nutrition, *your body can work* to its usual/customary workload, but the muscles keep firing and the respiratory system keeps functioning with less lactic acid build up (buffering). What people *learn* in hindsight is that what we think of as fatigue are actually the affects of sub-par/poor nutrition. Once adequate nutrition-density is provided with whole-foods, functional-foods and certain kinds of dietary supplements at certain times, we realize the muscles and cardiovascular system can be fatigued through duration of exercise, but continues to fire without delay...muscles that are malnourished feel tired and we think it's because we've reached our threshold...nothing could be further from the truth.

Offset genetic potentials:

When I talk about off-setting the genetic potentials, what I'm talking about is providing what I coined as the Basic Nutritional Building Blocks (B.N.B.B.s) [certain kinds of dietary supplements at certain times]. When the body consistently gets a wide spectrum of the fundamental nutritional components that aren't usually available consistently enough for active people, the signs, symptoms and other health idiosyncrasies we think we have to *learn* to live with can simply go away. I'm not talking about taking supplements to cure anything. I am talking about taking certain kinds of dietary supplements, at certain times, in order to give the cells the nutritional components which the DNA/RNA require, to carry out their blueprint *for health*, which food by itself/without dietary supplements isn't capable of providing active individuals.

Historically, the less nutrition the body gets the more seemingly inescapable health symptoms show up, but when people absorb enough nutrition the nagging health problems they thought they had to live with seem to go away. Some of the most-simple symptoms of sub-par nutrition are hands and feet that are often cold (commonly referred to as Raynaud's *Dis*-ease), unhealthy hair, skin and nails, frequent colds, flu/viruses, cravings/eating the same foods over and over, fatigue, over/under immune functioning and weight gain as well as chronic injuries that don't seem to heal very thoroughly.

If you're active, it just stands to reason that when *you feel better* and aren't having to deal with breathing problems, allergies, digestive problems and other chronic health problems your performance in training and exercise as well as recovery from training sessions and events is going to be more efficient.

It's not at all uncommon for people to have three or four health problems, that even if they are receiving treatment they think they have to live with them. But once they get their nutrition program *dialed-in,* the symptoms of the hereditary/genetic problems seem to go away. You could still say they have the genetic or hereditary potential, it's just that the signs and symptoms remain latent. With me personally, allergies, digestive problems and bleeding were how genetic/hereditary problems showed up in my health prior to proper nutrition. You *don't* necessarily *have to be suffering* with minor or major health problems while exercising, training and competing.

Chapter conclusion:

You really won't *know your true fitness* and athletic potential until you apply all three nutritional principles herein. The athlete who has their *nutrition* program *dialed-in* will outperform the naturally gifted athlete, every day. As far as fitness, fat-loss and general wellness, you'll get four times the results, in half the time by *applying* what I teach *herein.*

Let's talk about off-setting genetic/hereditary potentials.

Chapter Three

Off-setting Genetic/Hereditary Potential

Genetic-potential(s) or hereditary-condition(s) relates to health problems, signs, symptoms, syndromes and conditions, which left to their own or under the circumstances, where someone purposely or unwittingly withholds adequate nutrition, manifest as health problems.

Epigenetics:

As described on nature.com: *"Epigenetics involves genetic control by factors other than an individual's DNA sequence. Epigenetic changes can switch genes on or off and determine which proteins are transcribed."*

In simple terms, adequate nutrition (what I coined as the B.N.B.B.s) can provide the factors which the DNA/RNA uses to prevent unhealthy expression of genes or indirectly cause potential health problems/hereditary/genetics to remain [latent] "unexpressed" throughout life.

To further explain, in as simple as possible terms, people who have what they have been told are hereditary or genetic conditions, bad luck or otherwise unavoidable health problems, often *find* that when they get enough B.N.B.B.s for their particular body, health things they previously believed they had to live with simply become less intense or go *away* completely, for no apparent reason, improving overall quality of life and performance, but return once inadequate nutrition is inadvertently skipped or purposely discontinued

There's a ton of ongoing controversy on these kinds of topics, partly because each school of thought or profession has their own standards as well as informational biases that their profession adheres to. In other words, if *you* come from the world of treating *dis*-ease, there's the potential bias that information about preventing genetic *dis*-ease is invalid. Even in professional realms, people don't know what they don't know and would rather avoid giving any advice than advise they aren't sure of, which is responsible. For example, I read one study done out of Children's Hospital, Seattle that showed that unless a doctor or nurse has had success with what is considered adjunctive modalities, they don't share the information with their patients.

Because nutrition in general is misunderstood, even by health professionals, I've found there's *more mis*-information than valid information available and being shared within professional realms and among consumers...too much opinion and not enough correct application. There's a lot of money made from fake, bogus, hyped-up products that don't do anything good for the body. One of my specialties is to train people to get on a sensible, dietary supplement program to make up for inherent gaps in their daily nutrition habits. Even people who know really well how to *eat good* don't get consistent nutrition day-in and day-out...*knowing how you should eat is not the same as getting enough nutrition in your body.* People who know the most about nutrition take some supplements, even though they do eat really well every day, leaving nothing to chance...*no stone unturned*…filling in their nutritional gaps to maximize performance. If you leave stones unturned, your priorities might be mixed up and I would refer you to my other book again. This is a doing program, not a saying or "talking about" program....*doing.*

Some professionals say you don't have to *get enough nutrition* daily (that the averages over a period of time are enough for everyone), but, in my experience, rather than having an opinion or an idea (regardless of professional status), *body composition improvements* and blood chemistry lab results are the two most accurate, science-based ways to know if you're consuming enough nutrition as well as whether or not what you're consuming is getting onto your blood stream and into the cells where nutrition actually does its job...*putting food or supplements in your mouth and swallowing them* does not assure they're working (another reason why there's so much misunderstanding and mixed results with dietary supplements).

The point being that you can offset genetic, hereditary as well as health problems caused by medical treatment that could have been avoided. *You* don' have to suffer with nagging health problems, while *improving your performance*…in fact, nagging health problems indicate you're nowhere near your maximum performance level. Part of the reason being, that if you are bleeding or having any other type of emergency *you* should go to the emergency room, immediately. But, a large portion of the reasons why people go to the emergency room (about 90%) is from conditions caused by lifestyle factors (lack of proper exercise and nutrition), which *evolve* into chronic health conditions and ultimately become acute, emergency health conditions.

Case in point: Alberto Salazar;

Coach of Nike Oregon Project, American Track Coach, world-class distance-runner, author.

Alberto Salazar, author of *Alberto Salazar's Guide To Running and 14 Minutes: A Running Legend's Life and Death and Life* started out as a high school athlete and was a state cross country champion in 1975. From there, he went to the University of Oregon where he won numerous All American-honors, was a member of the 1977 NCAA cross-country championship team, won the individual NCAA cross-country championship in 1978, finished third in the Olympic trial 10,000 meter race to make the 1980 Olympic team. Alberto broke the 5,000-meter record in February 1981 at the Millrose Games in New York. His 13:22.6 beating the old record by nearly 20 seconds as he finished second.

From 1980-1982 Salazar won three consecutive New York City Marathons. Alberto excelled at distances from two miles to the 54-mile length of Africa's Comrades Marathon which he won in 1994 (the year the course went uphill).

At age 48 (June 30, 2007) and 158 pounds (144 being his competition weight) and approximately 5% body fat/still lean and running 25-30 miles a week, running six days a week, Alberto stopped breathing and dropped to the ground at the Nike Training Center in Oregon. *"They had to shock my heart four times before they finally got my pulse back, which was 13-14 minutes after I first went down"* said Salazar... *"Within an hour they placed a stent in a major artery."*

Prior, his doctor had noticed his blood pressure had been on the upswing for about a dozen years running about 140/97 (average normal would be about 120/80) and lowering to about 125/75 on medication. Alberto was also taking cholesterol medication, which lowered his total cholesterol to about 175.

Alberto had a complete physical, a couple-months prior to the event. He had seen his general practitioner who was really fit herself and had kept his health in check. Alberto even had an EKG performed and everything checked out fine, but he did have some family history of heart *dis*-ease. Ultimately, his doctor said it would have taken an exercise stress test to find the arterial blockage ahead of time.

Alberto's work ethic and workouts were legendary, going way beyond unconventional training to prepare his physiology for the stresses of competition, (some couldn't believe the intensity with which he trained), but in hindsight, Salazar said the component he neglected, even at his level of athletic development was the nutrition parts.

You can push the body which makes it "tougher" but to exercise doesn't keep the arteries cleaned out, especially with a genetic predisposition. In order to balance body chemistry, nutrition must be applied.

Let's talk about the structure of your program.

Chapter Four

Structure And Definitions

For simplicity in this book, when I refer to "workouts" I'm referring to any kind of exercise, training or fitness/athletic events you're doing or plan to do in the future. The point being that however and whenever you're physically, mentally & emotionally exerting yourself toward a goal(s) you'll have to *take proper exercise* strategy into account to prevent injury and make progress, as well as apply proper nutritional program principles: 1) Whole-foods 2) Functional-foods and 3) Certain kinds of dietary supplements at certain times.

Why my training style & information is fundamentally different:

I stuck around.

Today, there seems to be constant controversy about the "secrets" or the principles of fitness that work the best, get the fastest results, provide the most sustainable results and in the healthiest way possible.

It blows me away when I hear or see where trainers are promoting information that is long outdated ("calories-in, calories-out" for example). One of the upsides of personal training is that *you* can *become* a trainer with very little education, training or experience. The industry as a whole is regulated *very little*. The downside is that many trainers really don't know what they are talking about, let alone have ways to know they don't know *what* they're talking about!

Part of why what I teach and how I teach and how I go about *making sure of safety* and effectiveness are that I've been in the industry so long, that I learned where and when what I was promoting wasn't accurate nor effective. My training started out by having a personal trainer who really knew what she was doing and ***then I did exactly what she showed me to do, for weeks and months without skipping or changing anything.*** I *did the program exactly how she showed me to do it* and checked back with her any time I had a question to make sure I was doing the program correctly.

More often than not, clients hire a trainer, but then *pick* the program apart focusing on what seems convenient or by doing what won't interfere in their unfit/fat lifestyle. People *do the same thing* with information they get from their medical professionals (insist on the soonest possible visit, skip what their doctor tells them to do and then return later with the same complaint).

I have stayed in the industry long enough to find out what information stood the test of time. Many trainers drop out as soon as they realize they won't be earning a hundred-thousand-dollars, their first year. Most trainers don't stay in the industry long enough to find out what is *mis*-information and hype. How this shows up at the gyms is high turnover is personal training staff, meaning you may purchase training, but then the trainer you started out with isn't necessarily the trainer *you get personal training* from. Another reason for this dynamic is that gyms want sales people who they send through a three-day personal training seminar, so they can call them a trainer, whom can talk like a trainer (sound like a trainer) and once you purchase training, they place you with a different trainer to keep the 'sales' trainer selling.

The main reason I was so adamant about finding *what works* and what is hype, is because first and foremost I'm applying it to myself. If it doesn't work for me, it never makes it to my clients, as part of their program.

Outdated information:

To add to the hype information dynamic, many trainers are promoting outdated information that has been shown to be inaccurate, useless and even downright dangerous. All that stuff about starving yourself to lose weight, the magic diet pills and "no need to exercise" is still circulating. Just when you'd think the rumor is dead, it starts circulating as the newest, hottest thing again, igniting hope in people who don't know any better.

Trainers who don't care about the *long-term* health consequences continue to promote outdated and dangerous quick-fixes. There's a few reasons for this which I'll cover throughout the book. Quick-fixes sound promising and one way to know you're being suckered is if they say you don't have to do a *nutrition program* from the get go, offer the magic pill or imply exercise isn't important.

The money cycle:

The gym/fitness industry is big money. 80% of the population is overweight now and if you look at people who simply aren't fit, the numbers are pushing 95%. Having worked at some of the larger chains, I can tell you that some gyms look at the front door as an endless supply of people willing to put the money down, for their membership, but rarely use the facilities or equipment. Part of this is the consumer mindset...*that buying is getting and getting is having*. But, fitness being one of those things you can't buy no matter how much money you have...*it's a doing thing*.

But, people don't believe it. People convince themselves that they'll plunk down the money and *get fit* like those other people. A lot of people drop out, continue to pay their membership fee (because they're going to get started again next week), but skip the workouts and continue to gain more and more weight as each month passes. MOST people stop going to the gym within three-months of joining. Gym staff have seen so many thousands of people who join intending to get in shape, but simply don't follow through. So, having to watch out for their business, they move people through the motions of signing up, another portion of members buying personal training and still dropping out (gym keeps the membership fees, keeps the personal training fees and doesn't have to pay their trainers for training they didn't do)...*so it's quite a cash cow*.

I even asked a personal trainer manager at a gym on Capital Hill, Seattle why he was so mean and cold to the members and clients and he said, *"...because it doesn't matter, with the TV commercials there's an endless supply of people."* No matter how bad he treats them people keep coming in and *bringing* their *friends*, to plunk down the money thinking spending the money will show *results*, in fitness.

With the people who do *follow through* and *do* their *exercise* and nutrition program, they *get excellent results*, get in *amazing shape* and the new members see them thinking it's all about signing up and being around the equipment...*nothing to do with what they do*. Once the newbies realize they have to work to *get the results*, they get tired because their nutrition program is so weak, their motivation drops off and they drop out until next year's New Year's Resolution comes around *again.*

Gyms and their employees recognize the 90-day cycle the majority of the population participates in. Trainers provide information that causes their body to initially lose "weight"/they look smaller, their clothes fit more loosely, their friends (within month two and three) want to know the 'secret' and then they come into the gym wanting the secret...never realizing that that "kind" of weight loss is neither healthy nor sustainable and will likely be gained back by the fourth or fifth month.

By the third month, without a proper nutrition program, e.g. (1) Whole-foods 2) Functional-foods and 3) Certain kinds of supplements at certain times), motivation wanes, results have reached a plateau and the member has begun to gain back the unhealthy weight loss as well as more weight. But, by this time the first set of friends is in their second month of unhealthy weight loss and their friends have joined and the cycle continues...for a lot of gyms and trainers, it's not about maintaining clientele, but rather capitalizing on the next wave of "three-monthers" who *walk through the door.*

At smaller independent (non-chain), local studios where you're likely to be dealing with the owner/operator themselves or trainer who emphasizes education. That 90-day newbie dynamic is less likely since their business is based on maintaining clientele. *You* still have to *apply* a clear way *to know* if you're *getting healthy* results (body composition & blood chemistry), which I cover throughout my books, but hopefully if your health isn't improving and you're not feeling better, you wouldn't *continue* anyway.

Part of how gyms/trainers continue the 90-day cycle of repeated mistakes is to [not] give you copies of *your workouts,* nor write down anything about your workouts in *hope* of creating dependence on them. They walk you through a workout, but don't teach you how to think for yourself, as far as exercise program design nor nutrition planning. Nearly three-decades as a professional trainer has taught me that sustainable health & fitness is based on *taking correct actions,* consistently enough to get healthy results, then learning *how you did it* and then making decisions about how you spend your time, energy and resources to *continue* the processes in the future. Gyms know that they make way more income from the members who begin, stop, procrastinate and then *repeat over and over* than people who *succeed within the first three-months.*

With me, my initial trainer (Tracy), wrote everything down from the *beginning* and insisted I do the same. Every single workout I *checked off* what I *completed* as well as recorded/showed what I *missed* in any given workout. What this did was show me the patterns of a properly designed program, the progress of *consistency* and when it was time for a new workout (every six to eight-weeks).

Check your work!

Most importantly, the majority of trainers don't know for sure how to check if they program they designed for a client *is working* or not, let alone how to change what they're *doing* if the client isn't *getting healthier,* burning fat and gaining lean mass (accountability: body composition and blood chemistry).

Without knowing how to check their work, there isn't any accountability on the trainer's part and the client doesn't develop any accountability to themselves. Essentially, the trainer, in these cases hopes the client keeps training with them [simply for the sake of having a personal trainer], regardless of *results.* Often trainers *take* such brief certification courses they don't learn how to check their own *work.* Similar to mathematics, if you don't *learn* to check your work you'll miss points on the exams. In fitness-land, missing points means less than optimal health, slow if any weight loss and often a loss of lean mass...plateaus in *progress* followed by gaining weight back and often injuries.

So, some of the things that are *different* about my approach is that I know exactly how to get clients the *results* they *want,* how to improve their overall health in the process, how to *adjust course* if the initial plan wasn't working good enough (for me) and how to interpret the body composition numbers when we check body composition once a month (there are eight different variations in body composition you'll see when you check your body composition). A lot of trainers don't know what to do with all the variations and will simply try to push for a greater restriction in calories, to decrease body fat (when the client has already been restricting calories, the first three-months, there's no room to restrict anymore and definitely compromises health, let alone further sabotages further progress).

Let me make absolutely clear, as I will throughout the book that the only ways to know if the time energy and resources *you're investing* in your program are paying off are to (the first of each month) 1) Check your body composition 2) Check your resting heart rate + target heart rate and 3) Check/adjust your calorie requirements.

There's no exception, unless you're just going through the motions.

EVERYONE hits plateaus in fitness progress. If you don't *do these things from the beginning* then you won't know what has to change/improve in month three, four, five and so on.

If you don't do these things from the beginning then you won't know what has to change/improve in month three, four, five and so on.

At its best, the point of fitness training is to *learn* about your body, so you know how to make decisions about your program on a monthly basis, but more importantly, you learn to see how the decisions you make from moment-to-moment are either amplifying the results of your workouts and *nutrition* or sabotaging them.

The clients who want the program done "to them" are saying they don't want to be accountable or responsible, for making poor decisions and by not learning about those three points you do, the first of the month, ignorance remains bliss, but progress is inconsistent to say the least. Information and tracking things is nice, but if you don't know what to do with the information, it's pointless...it still comes back to what you're doing.

Any personal training you get should be educationally-based for the purpose of *empowering you* to *establish* a base line of proper habits (exercise AND nutrition), by which to compare all your future choices. If a trainer isn't having you write down or somehow document what you are doing with each exercise and nutritional choice, they're doing the training to help themselves, not with the primary outcome to help you know how to make choices for yourself.

Without *knowledge of yourself*, what worked and why, nothing you're doing will be sustainable...no one gets personal training forever.

Safety first!

First and foremost, the single greatest factor to consistent and *sustainable results* is creating a program that is safe (for your current level of fitness). If your program isn't designed to take your current level of conditioning into account, you'll likely "unexpectantly" get hurt and have to stop working out. It happens all the time. More often than not, injuries occur when people talk about wanting an exciting or sexy workout program that looks interesting or fun, but far exceeds their fitness level. A long-time friend of mine refers to this phenomena as "jacking-yourself-up" where, whether it's due to workouts that are too long (duration), excessive weight being used (intensity), excessive speed of a movement (ballistics), sloppy form or a combination of many factors.

It's very common for people to *get* personal training, but within the first three-months consider themselves experts and add exercises into their routine which they are not prepared for and hurt themselves. I recently had a client who was in her 50's and had never exercised in a structured way. On top of this, she insisted on skipping *the three-parts of nutrition.* She took it upon herself to add in advanced exercises, which I intentionally left out of her program, based on injuries and current fitness levels. Even though she was very consistent with her 3x/week program, by the third month her motivation and energy level was waning, aches and pains were showing up and by her fifth month she had completely quit, due to back pain. You see, its not at all uncommon for new clients to think because they are paying a trainer, that they know better than the trainer and go outside what was suggested, only to hurt themselves, inhibiting their ability, to exercise at all. Most of this is related to skipping the three parts of nutrition, which *enable clear thinking and motivation.*

When this happens, injuries can often be complex in nature, meaning not only is a muscle or tendon injured but the neurological factors are involved in such that even after the tissues heal, dysfunctional movement patterns remain. If an advanced athlete has an injury, more often than not, its related to weakness somewhere else in the body, combined with *emotional states related to* letting go, *moving forward and success* itself.

So, one of the most important reasons to seek help from an experienced and well-educated trainer is to design a program that *you are* currently prepared to perform/based on your current fitness level. Part of the reason I got such good results, from the get-go, during the first three-months of my own workouts, was because Tracy designed the program for me and [I followed it just as she told me and showed me, no exceptions, no changes, no eliminating the parts which could have seemed difficult or inconvenient]. A big factor in any fitness & nutrition program is doing novel and unfamiliar behaviors so you're *getting better results*...that's the point.

The ideas of a responsibly designed training program (regardless of your goals) is that it be and should include:

● Safe (prevents injury) designed with your current fitness and conditioning level,

● Somewhat *exciting* (novel, unfamiliar & challenging),

● Prevent over-training (*don't exercise too often*),

● Prevent too much intensity from workout-to-workout and throughout the year,

● Prevent too much volume (total number of sets, reps, etc.),

● Prevent too much frequency (don't exercise too often/*allow for maximum recovery between workouts,*

● Prevent random/pointless movements (e.g. activity/work is not necessarily exercise; the body adapts to movement, so doing the same things all the time does not provide ongoing benefit),

● Maximize efficiency (get the most done in the least amount of time). If you do incorrect action or what others are doing, *you* simply won't get the results you could. Hint, hint...exercise infomercials use professional fitness models! That's why people don't *get the results* promised from infomercial exercise programs...lots of jumping around, but little effectiveness!

● Prevent frustration (see beginning results within three days and then have ongoing improvements),

• Leave some gas in the tank (e.g. don't workout to exhaustion, ever time),

• *Produce measurable results* and consistent improvements and

Include all three parts of the thorough and complete nutrition program:

1) Whole-foods

2) Functional-foods and

3) Certain kinds of dietary supplements at certain times.

Leave some gas in the tank:

Most people who don't know any better workout until they've used up all their energy and then go home, and withhold food hoping they will get faster results by starving themselves. This is backwards-thinking and detrimental to health and any sustainable progress.

Properly designed and executed programs give the body a 'hint' of what direction you want *your body* to go in (burn fat, gain lean mass, gain strength, improve endurance, injury resistance)...meaning enough exercise (stimulation), to *let the body know what you want it to do*, then stop short of exhausting it...-*enough, but not too much.*

A significant portion of people who approach me for help who have already been working out but not getting the results they want are [doing too much] and [consuming too little nutritionally] and focusing on training their strengths, rather than improving their weaknesses, leaving them vulnerable to chronic injuries. You have to *leave some energy in your body,* at the end of the workout, and I'll tell you how to do this.

If you don't leave some energy in the body at the end of the workout, you'll end up doing too much too often with too little recovery ending up overtraining (a physiological phenomena where the body begins breaking down from doing too much, too often; *the three nutrition principles of a complete nutrition program buffer the overtraining affect, effectively reducing the risk).*

Knowing how to *eat correctly* or knowing you should *eat better* is not a substitute for sensible supplementation. Even people who know how to eat optimally have gaps in their diet that show up in how their body looks and performs. No one eats correctly all the time...not even me...I take certain kinds of supplements at certain times to *make up for the gaps in my diet*...it just makes sense and *produces better results* healthier body composition and healthier blood chemistry results than food alone.

Even people who start out well on their program *get good results* the first three to six months end up overtraining, getting injured and start going backward because as your fitness level increases, nutrition requirements increase...so as you progress through your workout programs, you increase your nutritional requirements incrementally... *because as your fitness level increases, nutrition requirements increase*...commonly accidentally overlooked or purposely skipped the outcome is the same.

By placing *emphasis on recovery* (rest and nutrition), you'll likely find you can *train more consistently* and feel better as time goes on rather than feeling and requiring more sleep as time goes on. Many people find that the amount of sleep they require (regardless how much they workout) is actually a symptom of malnutrition (one or more of the three nutrition principles).

Pros know:

Jim Wendler is a three-time letter winner at the University of Arizona (football) and has squatted 1000 pounds, in competition. In the 275-pound weight class, also performed 675-pounds in the bench press, 700-pound in the dead lift, and a 2,375 total pounds.

In the past, Jim taught classes on how to get that kind of strength. People insisted they wanted to do what he did, but when he talked about *"leaving some in the tank"* eager students consistently did more and more in their workouts (intensity, volume, duration), but skipped or removed the program parts related to recovery. Then people would complain they weren't getting the results they wanted!

Jim said, *"My response? You don't need to operate at your max to increase your max...guys are building muscle, avoiding burnout, and most importantly, making progress every workout. None of this is exactly revolutionary. I learned this in my freshman year. I've always made my best gains when I left just a bit in the tank."*

Chapter conclusion:

The first 90 days are critical to your success. If you cut corners, attempt quick-fixes, skip any of the three-parts of the nutrition program or change anything you'll miss the boat and likely wonder why. It's easier to not do what need to be done and that's why 80% of the population is overweight...*it's easier not to do the thing.*

80% of the results you get or miss out on from your exercise program is related to the three nutrition principles...*skip one or two parts and you'll miss the mark.*

Those three nutrition principles are so important to safety (people who skip these three nutrition principles get injured more often) and continued success that after the first cycle (however much is decided on in the beginning [up to three-months]) if someone isn't applying them the way I want them to, I release them, to go be trained by someone else. Part of what people get from me is a trainer with 30-years experience, with nutrition and the flip side is that as a client you have responsibility and accountability, also. If you want to pick a program apart, simply find a trainer who doesn't know any better and do a half effort from the get go...save us both time and make room for the people who do want to be shown what to do and how to do it and follow through on their commitment rather than making excuses...you won't use me to justify your excuses, but there's plenty of trainers who will gladly accept your money and watch you *not* follow through. Getting amazing results requires a lifestyle change, plain and simple.

Let's talk about the most common problems and solutions.

Chapter Five

The Next 90 Days:
The Seven Most Common Problems & Solutions

1. The single greatest factor that will provide or rob you of the results you earn during your workouts and structured recovery is waiting, procrastinating or flat out skipping, one or more of the three nutrition principles:

    1) Whole-foods,

    2) Functional-foods and

    3) Sensible supplementation: *certain kinds of supplements at certain times.*

2. Skipping adequate instruction:

Regardless of your goals in life or the area of endeavor, you have to get instruction, so you don't waste time or get hurt during the learning curve. In nearly three-decades, I've never seen a person know how to successfully develop their own program, even if they have historically been athletic or fit without study, instruction, training or all of them combined. You can develop instincts, which is preceded by correct action/habit, which is preceded by correct knowledge, which is preceded by correct instruction.

Without professional help you're wasting your time, energy and resources. If you have a good trainer you'll hear yourself saying something like, *"It was worth every penny and more...I'd do it again."*

If you get a poorly educated trainer who wants to train you, but doesn't want to teach you anything, search for a new trainer until you find the one who is a match. Let them know you want to learn how to workout not just be told what to do. Learn to discern correct knowledge and strategy from hype or outdated information.

3. Not measuring your body composition from day one:

Behind the three nutrition components, the most common overlooked factor for exceptional results and continued success is knowing where you are starting from, whether you are making progress on a monthly-basis and what to do once you have your body composition results.

Body composition determines how much you need to eat and what you need to adjust in your workouts to make progress and tells you if all the time, energy and resources are being invested or wasted.

If you don't know where you're starting from, there's no way to design a program properly and continued success (beyond three-months is unlikely).

Most of the time, clients say something like, *"Oh, I just want to get going, I'll do that later"*. People don't understand that there's no, *"...just get going,"* you're either on track from the beginning or not.

"Haste makes waste":

You may have heard me talk about the "hurry up and procrastinate" phenomena. Its where people work really hard at getting really fat and unhealthy, then make a quick emotionally-based decision to start exercising, are in a hurry to get going even pressuring their trainer to hurry up, then as soon as they get their program they start taking it apart disassembling the professionally designed program, skipping this, throwing this out and etc. The second thing that gets thrown out (second to nutrition) that assures failure is not learning to track your body composition (ratio/percentage of body fat to lean mass). If you don't know where you're beginning, no program will be designed specifically for you...it will simply be random activity that won't produce sustainable or measurable results...*frustration.* Even the unhealthiest, most dangerous program will cause a change in physical appearance and the way clothes fit for the first couple-months.

4. Wandering from the fundamentals:

One of the most common faux pas people unwittingly make, in the development of the workout programs, and/or getting started or back on track is jumping ahead too quickly. What this means in practical terms is that your personal fitness/conditioning level can't be faked. You can neither speed the fitness process up nor cut corners by attempting a program that is more complex, challenging or sophisticated than were your conditioning level is.

It's very common for people to join a gym, start going and then watch what other people are doing...especially the fit members and conclude they're going to do what they are seeing others do and get the level of results those people currently have.

What the majority of the population misunderstands is that some of the most fit people we see got that way by mastering basic exercises and programs and then doing them over and over...mastering them, over months and years. When we see people doing fast, heavy or complicated moves, exercises or circuits that look really fun, more often than not they have included these kinds of exercises into their basic program either for variety during a period of active recovery (lower intensity, more variety, less duration, less frequency), in order to stay active, but prevent over training and injury from doing too much too often. What happens is that we see someone who looks really fit and erroneously conclude that they got that way by doing the exercise we saw them doing, at that moment!

There's also the phenomena when gyms offer classes (HIIT, core, cycling, yoga, Pilates, mamba-jamba, etc.), in order to offer variety of amenities to members, but again, the point being to increase the number of members (increase their marketability among competing gyms) not necessarily are those classes going to get you the results you or any majority of the population insist you want (fat-loss, gain lean mass, gain strength, improve endurance)….justifying paying, but not going.

In the beginning phases of getting fit or coming back from a lay-off, you should be focusing on very basic exercises to build up basic muscular strength, tendon and ligament strength, flexibility, some balance and some cardiovascular conditioning to train your body to burn fat for energy rather than storing fat. This initial program should be performed for six to eight-weeks. I'm assuming you are working out three-times, each week with a day off, in between each workout for rest (e.g. M,W,F or T, Th, Sat.)...any more or less and you'll either over train or not get results.

Once you have done a basic resistance and cardiovascular training program for six to eight-weeks (18-24 workouts), you've gotten about as much adaptation as you can from that particular program, at that particular time. An important point I want you to take away is that the adaptation process (getting fit/getting results from your program) comes from doing a certain set of exercises again and again, with some rest between each workout (the recovery time). The people who don't get satisfying results from their program are often switching their exercises up so often the body doesn't go through the process of adaption (getting stronger and gaining endurance) from the program itself. [The people who say they get 'bored' practicing the fundamentals are telling you they have psychological barriers they haven't addressed yet].

You have to do a set of exercises a number of times to determine your starting strength for those exercises and establish good, safe form, go through the process of gaining as much strength and endurance from those particular exercises and then mastering your form and pushing to get the most from those particular exercises before moving on (this process typically takes six to eight-weeks).

During each eight-week phase, your primary goal is to use as much weight as you can for the suggested repetition (rep) range, while maintaining safe form to prevent injury...a balance between pushing to use heavier weight on each rep while maintaining safe form and range of motion (ROM).

By consistently sticking to the fundamental exercises in phases (periods) you'll get better, faster and more noticeable/measurable results than attempting exercises, which seem more fun and stimulating to your mind, but are too advanced for your body to benefit and/or from doing too much variety in any given six to eight-week period. Once you have established a very solid base of exercise experience (six months or more) you can reasonable begin adding more complicated, challenging, more intense, faster, exercises while relying on the fundamentals as your base plan (continue with fundamentals, but add variety on the side).

Like most things in life, what we want to do (or think we'll do) and what we need to do to reach our goals are two different things. Much of the information, videos, etc., we see in media is really geared toward intermediate and advanced level workouts, not beginners. The faster the movements the more dangerous for the unconditioned person (for the joints and pre-existing injures). The faster the movement the more power required by the tissues and the more power required the higher the likelihood of injury or trouble recovering from the injury.

The intermediate and advanced program won't necessarily produce satisfactory results in the beginner and are very likely to get you injured since the tendons, ligaments, bones and joints haven't gone through enough adaptation to be fit/conditioned/strong enough to respond to the more advanced exercises (meaning the stress is placed too much on the joints and connective tissues than on the muscles and how they relate to one another). Additionally, the nervous and hormone systems have to be conditioned and adapt to workloads too...so going too fast isn't more effective and likely causes injury. If the core and postural muscles haven't had time to come back online (become active), injuries to the neck, low-back and knees are likely, as described earlier.

If you don't begin with and stick to a basic-program, you'll be disappointed with the results you get and potentially hurt yourself. By sticking to a solid, professionally designed program and following through on the three-parts of a good nutrition program you'll get better results than you've gotten before and most likely better results than any of your friends have or are getting.

A big part of getting great, measurable, noticeable results is simply having the drive to show up for your workouts and being patient and consistent enough to allow the program to affect you.

My clients begin seeing and feeling benefits from their workouts within about three-days (assuming they do exactly as I ask without changing nor leaving anything out). That's how effective this simple program can be.

5. Doing too much too often:

You would think that most people miss out on results from not doing enough. In the first three-months, this is true...most people quit their program, within the first three-months.

If people make it through the first three-months, especially if they haven't gotten really good results, they often start making up reasons in their heads why that is. [It's usually related to the three-parts of nutrition, but most people make up other reason, in their head]. More often than not, people conclude 'more is better'. Meaning whether they initially got good results or not, as they continue skipping the three fundamentals I teach you have to do the first of every month: (1) Recalculate resting heart rate (RHR) and target heart rate (THR), 2) Recheck body composition (body fat level) and 3) Recalculate caloric requirements), they get further away from their goals, while being inconsistent with nutrition.

Each of those three things you check the first of each month assures you're moving toward your goals and maintaining the progress you've made, without getting off track wasting time, energy or money.

If you don't recheck those three things the first of each month, you won't know if what you're doing is working or not. Ideally, a professional trainer/coach would insist these three things are rechecked, the first of each month, to assure ongoing success and/or to help you get back on track before too much time, energy and money has been lost in ineffectiveness.

When these three things aren't checked, any workouts or nutrition activities are random...they aren't based in reality...that means you spent time, energy and money and got nothing or even went backwards. The key point here is that the people who get the best results are the ones whose attention to details is consistent...*it's the consistency to basics that yields seemingly phenomenal results*...the kinds of results where people say, *"Whoa, what have you been doing?!!"*

BUT, when people don't track those three key points, the first of each month, they usually conclude they aren't doing enough workout and eating too many calories...which is the opposite of what you should be thinking. So, usually, typical people go through a three to nine-month period (months four through twelve) of doing too much and eating too little and outright skipping the functional-foods and certain kinds of supplements at certain times, leaving them over trained, drained and depleted. Even the most-inept trainee will realize nine-months is too long to go, without progress.

By the time they do contact a trainer (if they do at all) they are malnourished and exhausted wondering, *"What happened?...I'm doing more and more, but I feel like I'm going backwards!"* Then, being malnourished, they want to debate the concept of nutrition, as their body continues to be malnourished!

Recovery, recovery, recovery!

Just as important as doing enough exercise often enough is resting (recovering) enough to allow your body to respond to your workouts. Workouts essentially (if designed and executed properly) give your body a message (to the nervous system and hormone systems) of what direction you want to go in (your goals) and then the body should respond by adapting to the activity (stimulus) and nutritional building blocks you're putting in: 1) Whole-foods 2) Functional-foods and 3) Certain kinds of supplements at certain times. Neither of these three are optional.

Because your body's ability to respond to the workouts is dependent on recovery and nutrition, without enough of either you simply won't get the results as quickly nor as thoroughly as you want. If you do get some initial results, they won't be maintainable/sustainable, by trying to do so with food alone. **In fact, about 80% of the results you do get or [miss out on] are related to your nutritional status.** A key point here to memorize and tell your friends is that the single greatest factor the permits/maximizes recovery between workouts is the quantity, quality, consistency and timing of nutrition. If you skip any of the three-parts of nutrition, you'll leave gaps in your nutritional program, which inhibit maximum performance of your body. Food alone won't provide enough nutrition-density to meet the demands of working out and a good indicator trainers use to know whether clients take their health seriously is their attitudes about certain kinds of dietary supplements at certain times. *Apathy produces regret.*

The people who don't take their long-term health seriously always skip supplements or take a low quality supplements that don't even produce any results, just to say they are taking something. How trainers choose which clients to maintain and which ones to let go are the ones who follow through and leave no stone unturned, don't cut corners nor make excuses for not following through. If you skip quality supplements (one third of the nutrition program) you're doing all the work and getting partial results. You have to put gas in your car, air in your bike tires and nutrition in your body.

6. Resistance-training before cardio:

Again, a very common phenomena in the gym scene is when people are convinced they want to do their cardio/aerobic workouts prior to resistance-training. In short, in order to get results from your workouts, do the resistance/weight training first followed by whatever cardio, aerobic or endurance training you intend to do.

In short, the ways the body uses energy, if you do the cardio, aerobic or endurance training you intend to do first, the energy needed within the muscles is no longer available (it got used up in the cardio/aerobics). Often, people unwittingly doing cardio first will complain of feeling nauseated, weak or too tired to do the resistance-training afterward...*symptoms of depletion.*

When I was a trainer at Gold's Gym, Capital Hill, Seattle I overheard a member telling his friend he didn't feel good. His friend asked, *"Why?"* and his friend said he had, *"... done cardio before weights and that always happens."* His friend said, *"You're supposed to do your weight training first."* And the guy replied, *"Yay, but I like to do cardio first."* So, even though he always feels sick from the way he structured his workouts, he still liked doing it that way? -*You tell me.*

There is a common phenomena today where people feel the need to make independent (emotionally-based) decisions, even though the results of the decisions are detrimental to their short-term goals, as well as their long-term health. Sometimes its referred to as anonymity or independence...people have the right to a point to make poor decisions and experience the consequences of those choices!

In order to burn fat, gain lean mass, gain strength and improve endurance (and after a brief warm up) do your heavy work, first (resistance-training, weight training, core, etc.), then progress to your fat-burning cardio, cardiovascular-conditioning and high-intensity cardiovascular-training, following the resistance-training (depending on your goals).

By doing it in this [order] you'll notice your strength improving much more quickly and you'll feel better during your cardio work. If you don't have the energy to do cardio after resistance-training, either too much overall workout is being done (volume) or you aren't in good enough shape to do that much resistance and cardio (current fitness level) or your nutrition is inadequate (lack of fuel, preparation or recovery) or, all things being equal you aren't focusing on your motivation.

The cardio part should be lower intensity than the resistance-training, so it's almost like an extended cool down period from the resistance-training. Aim for 50 minutes of resistance-training followed by 20 minutes of fat-burning cardio...*that's it*. If you still don't think you have the energy for both, do much lighter weights, focusing on full range of movement and form, so you have more energy during cardio until your body builds up adequate fuel from your nutrition habits.

People who reverse the order and do cardio first are often surprised that after weeks or months of workouts, they have gained fat and lost lean mass, lost strength, decreased endurance and have begun experiencing the effects of overtraining and malnourishment (doing too much, eating too little and withholding certain supplements at certain times/lack of nutrition-density).

7. Failing to learn there are three main types of aerobic workouts:

There's 1) Fat-burning cardio (low intensity) 2) Cardiovascular-conditioning (medium intensity) and 3) VO2 training (high intensity). Sport-specific activity depends on which sport you're preparing for.

With eighty-percent of the population overweight now, most people who seek personal training are looking to burn fat to some extent. Even competitive athletes want to dial-in their strength-to-weight ratio for their specialty. Fat-burning cardio is just that: lower-intensity aerobic-training that has been set up based on your resting heart rate (RHR) and adjusted for you age tends to tap into fat and use it while preserving the carbohydrate and protein you need to have healthy lean mass and build the basis of your metabolism (calorie burning).

True, there's controversy about this but as always, I don't rely on pet-theories, or the "workout-of-the-month" that seems fun and sexy. The reason I know this works is because I insist on checking body composition, heart rate and calorie requirements, the first of each month...remember? Are you reaching your overall outcomes?

By rechecking your RHR the first of each month, you readjust the target heart rate zone you're working in during cardio workouts...based on your latest fitness level. No matter what workout you do your body will adapt to the workload, but adaptation does not equate to continued progress...adaptation just means the workouts get easier and you can do higher intensity work.

But, more prematurely adding intensity isn't necessarily going to help you reach your intended goals. You still have to workout within your fitness level (indicated by your resting hear rate), otherwise most people (left to their own) do too much intensity in order to reach their goals (more is not better). The bright side is that even at the lower intensity fat-burning zone, you'll still be adapting and becoming more fit with each month that passes...doing too much too soon or going too hard in the beginning usually backfires, since it doesn't take your current fitness into account. People who do too much too soon don't stick around because they are working outside their level of fitness and burn themselves out, rather than allowing the body to adapt...you can't force the body to become fit, after time/years of disuse and it doesn't matter if you previously were fit...it takes time. In fact, in the UK a new *dis*-ease has been identified, named Stone Syndrome, which is when people in their 40's who haven't been consistent, with their workouts begin exercising, but in the absence of adequate nutrition and ability to recovery from their workouts, get injured and develop a whole host of problems, from attempting to progress too quickly, in attempt to make up for lost time (named for actress Sharon Stone).

The single greatest factor that makes progress happen faster is the three points of nutrition: 1) Whole-foods 2) Functional-foods and 4) Certain kinds of dietary supplements at certain times, from day-one!

You can't outrun poor nutrition-density with any amount of exercise, but your body will respond more quickly, more thoroughly and the results you'll get will be more sustainable, by applying the three-nutrition points, from the get go. I screen who I'll accept as a client and after the first month or so, if the client wants to continue have me, but skip important steps I simply refer them to a trainer/coach who doesn't provide accountability or hold the clients accountable. After decades of this, I can pretty much predict who will reach and maintain their goals and which ones will do some work but then complain they aren't getting results even though its related to them not doing what they agreed to do...*people believe they will get results even though they are skipping steps....but, wonder why they have never reached their goals before!*

What's really sad is when people lose a bunch of "scale weight" simply, by decreasing food intake (inadvertently decreasing nutrition-density) and increasing activity level (which increases the body's nutritional requirements) and then as they get close to their goal their body stops losing fat, health problems start showing up and they insist they don't know why...they're smarter than their trainer!

As you get more fit, your nutritional requirements increase. Purposefully withholding 1) Whole-foods 2) Functional-foods and/or 3) Certain kinds of dietary supplements at certain times, always backfires, it's just a matter of time. I'm not the type of trainer to force clients to do what they need to do, I simply won't keep them on as a client if they sorta' sweep my suggestions under the carpet, as if they don't know any better or that the know better than their trainer. The benefit of having a trainer with so much experience is that I'm paying attention...the down side is that *I'm paying attention.*

Because I do so much social-media, have so many books published, do so much public-speaking, etc., I get more requests from potential clients than I can work with. Its not at all uncommon for people to read my books, contact me, insist they want me as their trainer, but then as soon as we talk they begin back-peddling, side-stepping and attempting to weasel out of the five-parts of a complete program. Most often, people try to get out of the nutrition, even though I tell them its not optional, from the get-go. In these cases, I won't work with them. I work with the people who want a step-by-step, all-encompassing program...not a picked apart program that doesn't work. In cases where people do begin with me, but try to back out on my nutrition suggestions, I discontinue them, as a client. I only have room for so many client-hours, per week and I prioritize the people who apply my nutrition strategies, from day-one.

Fat-burning cardio:

Fat-burning cardio consists of alternating between 60% and 70% of your max heart rate throughout the cardio workout (considered low-intensity). Low-intensity, a relative term, because each month you get more fit and the zone changes to reflect your new fitness level and to maintain fat-burning progress. Later, I'll give you the formula for dialing in your own target zone for maximizing your fat-burning cardio.

Heart conditioning cardio:

Although there is improvement in heart conditioning from even the lower intensity aerobic conditioning, to target the heart to be more prepared for endurance events like running, cycling, swimming and rowing, part of your cardio workouts would be in the 70% - 80% heart rate range.

Part of the distinction here is that if you intend to do those kinds of events like running and cycling, you'll be a lot better off focusing on getting your body fat level (body composition) reduced to 10% to 15% (or lower), before beginning heart/cardiovascular conditioning. The reason being is that having body fat higher than 20% indicates some insulin-resistance going on...that means your body is storing fat, but not tapping back into it to use it as energy...ineffective energy storage and use/poor performance. Insulin resistance encourages atrophy and poor recovery.

If you've heard the idea of 'spot reduction' where a person tends to store fat on the hips or stomach this is the result of insulin-resistance...doing aerobic-training, but still have excess body fat. If you frequent events like 5k races and fun runs and such you'll see people who seem active and fit but they're still fat...a symptom of a malformed workout program. Not only is the excess fat bad for your health, its adding weight to your frame (stored energy) that can't be used during the event itself. The result is that your body isn't making the best use of energy.

[Each pound of excess fat adds about four pounds of weight to the joints...think about it]. Each 1% of fat equals about 2 pounds of fat.

If you have excess body fat (more than 20%) and you're very active, it's kind of like you skipped the developmental step of training your body to burn fat and went right to cardiovascular-conditioning...you might be able to push your body to do more, but the concept of discipline and personal development come into play. You're effectively pushing your body to do more than it's conditioned to do and carrying more energy (in the form of fat) than you can make use of during the duration of your chosen athletic events. It only makes sense that a step in your fitness development was skipped. Go back and train to get your body composition reduced/dialed-in.

VO2 conditioning cardio:

In general, VO2 relates to very higher intensity workouts, like you'll see in the Winter Olympics where the Nordic skiers are going all out for long periods of time or the Tour deFrance. In everyday life VO2 doesn't have much practical application since the intensity of exercise required to improve it, versus the benefits you would experience on a day-to-day basis are low, meaning you could train for it, but the use of the benefits are low, during an average day for a non-athlete, or people who aren't soldiers or police/emergency/tactical personnel.

Some careers like professional athletics, law enforcement, EMS, military, etc., want to spend a fraction of their weekly routine in the VO2 zone, [but to do so frequently assures over training, burn out and injury]. This zone would mean going into 80% or more of your max heart rate intermittently and would require professional help figuring out where to plug it in to your workouts to get the most benefit and the least adverse effects.

Now, we'll get into how to set your goals.

Chapter Six

Identifying And Defining Your Goals

In continuing the conversation about how and where we trip ourselves up, and unwittingly sabotage our fitness goals, one of the primary places this happens is before we ever even begin performing the program itself.

You know from my previous book, *Weighting To Wait,* the emotional state(s) we *choose* to allow to occupy our mind and affect our *behavior* determines, from the get-go, how likely we are to experience *success* in the first three-months...and sets the stage for future success or lack thereof. It's also possible for the emotions to interfere with each level of progress, as our new level of fitness and athletic development conflict with old, outdated programming. Whether a you're new to fitness or moving up through the ranks of competition, a weekend 5k warrior or Olympic hopeful, there's always the potential for emotional states to need updating to match the new, higher aspirations.

The *"hurry-up and procrastinate"* cycle I talk about, is a form of impulsivity, where people go way too long, not working out or making sure their body gets the three keys of a solid nutrition program and then impulsively jump into random activity hoping they'll reach the goals that match the picture they hold in their mind, of what they want their future to be. A main reason why people don't *get the results* they want is because they have a picture in their mind of what they want to look like, or a feeling of *how they want to feel,* but then don't take the time to build a program that would get them those goals, nor hire someone to do it for them.

Like any skill in life, we have to learn information somewhere. The school-of-hard-knocks, also known as the learning-curve, is so steep in fitness and long-term health that most people won't get there without professional help, at least in the beginning. Even if you only get professional help every few months to *set your program up* you'll still be ahead of the curve compared to people who attempt to set up a program on their own.

The people you hear about who decide one day to *suddenly start* walking to lose weight and a year later they have lost a hundred-pounds, have effectively lost 'weight' but often the long-term affects of losing lean mass, bone density and lacking nutritional-density in their regime end up being smaller in general but still lacking long-term health (*you can't outrun poor nutrition with any amount of exercise*) and often end up with numerous *de*-generative *dis*-ease symptoms (the weight may be reduced, but internal health has not been attended to nor improved).

The people who have prior athletic experience come in with work ethic and a mindset of doing, but often have no idea how to *program* their own *success* outside the structure of their chosen sport(s). That's not a slam on athletes, but rather a testament to the benefits of structure...the more structured your program and the more consistently attentive *you* are to the different parts of your workout structure, the better and faster and more sustainable the results you get and *keep*, the better you'll *feel* and the *better* your long-term health.

Part of the reason athletic-types get so out of shape, so quick, outside the realm of their sport has to do with prioritization, peer-pressure and team environment.

When we chose to take part in a team effort, we know that if we don't *show up* for practice there will be consequences for not making the team effort a priority...*social pressure for letting others down...hint, hint.* Athletes know better than to let down those around them, by leaving a stone un-turned. If you skip a step, you're team will see the consequences of that decision.

When we don't respond to the expectations of the team, to contribute to our very best to the team, peer-pressure keeps us in the game...*present to the current goals....hint, hint.*

If we let the team down our behavior will be frowned on by people we made a commitment(s) to...*follow through or lack thereof....hint, hint.*

If we show up with a negative attitude, that won't be tolerated long either as attitude, whether positive or negative can affect everyone around as well...an open-minded, positive expectation and *looking-forward-to-a-bright-future,* coachable attitude vicariously lifts everyone up.

In these three examples, we can notice the common denominator... the thing that makes the difference...is simply showing up and doing some work. How much work you do on any given day depends how well you're taking care of your overall health (nutrition and recovery)...*how good you feel* on that particular day.

Regardless of how *you* think you *feel* leading up to a workout, you really won't know if you're *prepared* for a workout, until you've done five minutes of physical activity. If you've eaten enough calories and consistently put enough nutrition-density in your body, when you do five-minutes of activity, you should feel like a horse trying to get out of the starting gate.

Most of the lack of motivation or feeling like *you* don't have the energy to exercise today is emotional fatigue...which is relieved by...*yes, working out*. The common mistake today is concluding that how we 'feel' in the moment is the determiner of whether or not it will be worth it to work out today/tonight (temporary emotionally-based decision, affecting long-term results). Newbies have trouble separating physical fatigue, from emotional fatigue.

One of the ways seasoned trainers and coaches can predict who will be a good investment of their time is by listening intently to how people talk in relation to their workouts. The people who talk about working out or skipping workouts based on how they 'feel' emotionally aren't likely to follow through. The reason for this is that the day-to-day grind of life (if your emotional status is left to chance) can leave a person feeling bogged down, tired and foggy (also a side effect of subpar nutrition/skipping one or more of the three parts of nutrition)...the seeming opposite of what you would expect leading up to your workout(s).

The people who get amazing *results* from seemingly simple/basic workouts are the ones who acknowledge their emotional state (being present) and regardless of how they think they feel, go workout out anyway...knowing from experience that feeling emotionally bogged down is a symptom of either too much emotional energy being expended leading up to the workout or exposure to too much negativity from others, on a routine basis...hint, hint. Emotional feelings are not a true indicator of your readiness to work out, just like thirst is not an accurate indicator of hydration level of your body, nor are there many accurate indicators of poor nutrition.

An exception to this phenomena is people who are doing too much workout, too often. Over-training/depletion of the nervous and hormonal systems of the body (too much intensity, frequency or duration of exercise/training) is indicated by feeling emotionally-drained and accompanied by lack of motivation...the difference being how much you've been doing within the last three-months, followed by injury, most often the low back, shoulders and knees.

How to know for sure (if you're over-training) is to consistently check your resting heart rate (RHR) upon awakening in the morning, before getting up. Any average increase/rise in your RHR, as the months go by, indicates your body is being stressed by your workouts versus adapting to the workouts and noticing decreased heart rate that goes along with getting in better cardiovascular shape. If your heart rate in getting increasingly higher, you're stressing your body out and that would be a better indicator of whether you are emotionally bogged down or actually needing to lighten up your workout intensity or even take a week off to actively recover and come back stronger.

If you have been over-training in *hopes* of making up for lack of progress (from lack of progressive structure) you'll *notice* that by taking seven days off, you won't lose any gains you've made and will *notice* you come back *stronger* than before the week off (after the three parts of a complete nutrition program, recovery is priority number one).

Balancing your program design:

What most of the public wants is to reduce their body fat level, gain strength, gain some lean mass including healthy bone mass and *improve* their endurance, as well as become resistant to injury. If you're not or haven't been getting this from *your program*, then you're unwittingly doing 'random activity' versus carrying out a structured program based on *your goals*.

Needs of the body:

The ideal program is going to give you all the things above, but in addition you'll notice measurable improvements in your cholesterol levels, blood sugar, triglycerides, blood pressure, less aches and pains, more energy, more mental and emotional clarity, consistency and stability (less moodiness/swings) as well as reduction of symptoms, in those classes known as hereditary or genetic conditions. If you're going through the motions of a program and your blood chemistry numbers aren't improving, it most likely has to do with the quality, quantity and consistency of *nutrition-density* you put *in your body* or withhold from yourself ***(you can't outrun poor nutrition with any amount of exercise)***

...believing or telling yourself you don't see a need for nutrition doesn't make the need by your body for nutrition less real, it simply means you're in denial or haven't gotten serious about your commitment, yet..*an attitude problem.*

Instincts?

It's very common for people to *have a goal in mind* (fat-loss, lean mass, bone density, etc.) and then see an exercise program and think that by doing that program they'll reach their goals...it doesn't work that way...*thinking is not doing.*

By sticking to a basic program and focusing firs on nutrition-density: 1) Whole-foods 2) Functional-foods and 3) Certain dietary supplements at certain times, you'll begin to understand that exercise/activity/working out is the stimulus for the body to change. But, without the nutrition-density the body can't fully carry out the response to the stimulus. Until you get enough nutrition on board, on a consistent basis, you really won't have a clear standard by which to base future choices for your exercise programs. Without enough nutrition-density, your body isn't responding fully to any workouts you do.

Without full response, you don't understand what works and what doesn't. If you don't know what works and what is ineffective *for your body*, you never *develop* your fitness instincts. Without the three parts of nutrition, I'm doing my part to train you, but you aren't doing your part.

Instincts are developed by doing complete and thorough *correct action* consistently enough to notice what definitely works...if what you're doing is only half way/half effort you don't have anything to compare correct actions to, so you don't know what to do when your body hits a training plateau, like everyone does throughout their life.

By getting a *full response* to your workouts, you learn what to do in the future to *get* consistent, sustainable *results!*

So, by having a workout that is structured and consistent and by following through on the three-points of your nutrition program, you'll know when you re-check your body composition the first of every month, what the numbers actually mean. Had you skipped parts of the nutrition program, the numbers you get from re-checking your body composition and resting heart rate are based on a partially-nourished status, so any *changes* you make to your program are once *again* random activity.

Without being consistent with your nutrition you'll eventually (every six weeks to three-months) hit a plateau; stagnation sets in followed by frustration. What assures you'll get exceptional results from the time, energy and resources you invest in learning to workout properly is how consistent you are with the three parts of your nutrition program. The differences between the people who get so-so or no-no results and the people who get amazing results comes down to the three parts of nutrition.

Calories vs nutrition-density:

Getting enough calories to fuel your workouts is important, but the two single greatest nutrition factors are: 1) Eating low-glycemic foods to stabilize blood sugar and 2) Nutrition-density: (1) Whole-foods 2) Functional foods and 3) Certain dietary supplements at certain times).

Whether a person is eating too few calories or a few too many, it comes down to how those calories get process and assimilated and that process is dependent on nutrition-density and low-glycemic foods, to prevent swings in the blood sugar level, which triggers the release, of insulin.

A person could be eating too few calories by *eating low-glycemic* foods and getting enough nutrition-density and reach their goals or eat too many calories and still *get very lean* and strong and improve their endurance. A reason for this is that the main benefits people want (fat-loss, strength, lean mass & endurance) come down to the body chemistry being balanced and functioning efficiently. Whether you eat too many or too few calories, has little effect on the chemistry, unless nutrition-density is lacking: (1) Whole-foods 2) Functional-foods and 3) Certain dietary supplements at certain times).

This is part of the reason I don't tell people what foods they should eat meal-to-meal, day-in-and-day-out: During the first three to twelve months people who haven't had training are generally malnourished to begin with...their taste buds, cravings and sense of what's good and tasty is skewed...the more malnourished a person the more they unconsciously and emotionally place junk food, S.A.D.C.R.A.P., fast-energy foods & drink, into the makeup of their daily routine.

What I have found across-the-board, is that the more malnourished a person is the more they eat food and drink that is low in *nutrition-density* and insist they don't like nutritious foods. BUT, those who take certain dietary supplements at certain times, build up their nutrition-density *savings account* (in their body and brain) and they are unconsciously drawn to nutritiously-dense foods.

When people start 'forgetting' to take their supplements, like people do with their prescription medications then within two or three-months the cravings start back and the S.A.D.C.R.A.P. starts getting worked back into the diet...then they say they aren't feeling as good...they are missing workouts...and they, *"...don't know what happened..."*

The *brain* has ways of giving us sensations when the blood sugar is low...but the sensations for lack of nutrition-density *is* also the sensation of low blood sugar, lack of caffeine, etc. In other words, you might not have a sensation of malnutrition, but you'll see yourself grabbing junk food instead of whole-foods...that is the sign of subpar nutrition!

In other words, the people who get the best results, the most sustainable, maintainable results are the people who purposely seek and consume (1) Whole-foods 2) Functional-foods and 3) Certain dietary supplements at certain times) whether they 'feel' like it or not. These people have made the cognitive connections, that in order to get the results they insist they want they have to put the nutrition-density in even though the brain is indicating to eat sugar, junk fats, ice cream, alcohol and caffeinated substances.

Within the brain is the limbic system which helps to regulate blood sugar and emotional driven reactions (the hands grabbing S.A.D.C.R.A.P. and putting it in the mouth). Until a person becomes desperate enough (sick and tired of being sick and tired) to over-ride their emotionally *driven* consumption habits, they usually won't consider supplements. Until their desire to change exceeds their desire to stay the same or stay on the same path, they'll do and say anything to avoid taking supplements...*addictions show up like that. Cravings for healthy foods come back online.* A reason being that the consumption of the junk foods and fast energy foods are a quasi-coping mechanism for stress. If you take away the junk food coping tool before replacing it with (3) Certain dietary supplements at certain times, the person would have no way to deal with life's stressors.

This is a big reason (an one indicator of future success or failure) that I have my clients continue eating and drinking whatever junk food they are used to relying on for the first 30 days, while they are taking 3) certain kinds of dietary supplements at certain times, until their nutritional savings account builds up within their brain...-once the nutritional savings account builds up within the limbic brain (emotional eating and emotional based behavior) and then spills over to fill up the frontal cortex (where rational thinking and behavior occurs) then the desire, cravings or want for junk food, S.A.D.C.R.A.P., energy drinks, tobacco, alcohol and so forth simply go away...as the nutrition-density decreases for whatever reason, the cravings come back just like clockwork...it's consistent and predictable.

You can't really see these processes occurring inside the brain, per se, but you can tell how nutritionally fueled the brain is and to what extent by your behaviors. If you're *eating*, relying on and looking forward to or preoccupied with junk food, you don't have enough *nutrition-density* in your brain, it's that simple.

If you have lost all cravings for three months (not just using short term will-power) and they continue to stay away, then you likely have enough nutritional-density in your brain. If you 'forget' to take your supplements or tell yourself they aren't important anymore or whatever excuse you come up with and start to notice junk food distracting you again then you can estimate that your brain is getting low in nutrition-density (certain dietary supplements at certain times) again...*it's just a process that goes on as long as we live, like maintaining anything.*

So, instead of telling people what foods they 'should' be eating (insisting they want to be told what foods to eat: *a sure sign they don't intend to follow through*), since no one wants to be told what to eat nor eat foods they aren't nutritionally balanced enough to appreciate, I teach 'style' of eating, not which foods to eat.

Your main focus on style of eating should be a) Do nutrition-density first: (1) Whole-foods 2) Functional-foods and 3) Certain dietary supplements, at certain times) and b) Learn all about low-glycemic foods (which and how foods affect blood sugar). By stabilizing blood sugar levels, you're effectively training the body to become more sensitive to insulin, thereby training your body to burn fat and maximize lean mass instead of storing every calorie as fat.

The more you get your blood sugar in control, thereby stabilizing it, the results you get from your workouts will be greater, come faster and will be more stable.

The third part of the importance of nutrition is the 'timing' of nutrition-density (1) Whole-foods 2) Functional-foods and 3) Certain dietary supplements, at certain times) and low-glycemic food stuff.

Timing in relation to getting the best results from your workouts for the least time, energy and resources means: 1) Eating in advance of activity 2) Eating smaller amounts more frequently 3) Refueling with functional-foods post-workout, within the first and second hours after your workouts.

Reducing calories won't help you in the long run and will even cause fat gain, if the nutrition-density and glycemic factors aren't taken into account first. Reducing calories without increasing nutrition-density always backfires. Attempting to go cold-turkey, on junk food and S.A.D.C.R.A.P., before building up the B.N.B.B.s in your body and brain, also backfires. Not wanting S.A.D.C.R.A.P. is a function of a properly nourished brain, not artificial will-power. Let's talk about the four key questions.

Chapter Seven

The Four Key Questions
For Results And Continued Progress

A main reason so few people *get excellent,* sustainable *results,* from their exercise program, is that they don't know how to tell if (during the process of doing their program) the *program is working* (improving health, burning-fat and gaining lean mass, while improving blood chemistry).

There's thousands of programs for weight loss and fitness nowadays. They all promise the same things: *fast weight loss.* Whether its fat-loss, gaining lean mass, improving strength and/or gaining endurance these four key questions will let you know if the program is doing what its promised to do.

Most activities people do are distractions:

Fitness has to be an intentional, primary, lifestyle focus or there will be too many other distractions that get prioritized higher than fitness.

In most gyms, the whole point is to get the client to sign on the line (whatever you say your goal is, they imply you'll get it by joining). Most people quit after three-months because the program lacked accountability, the member avoided responsibility and lacked understanding and there was no standard developed to stay on track, let alone how to get back on track if the program doesn't seem to be working.

As a beginner or advanced trainee, your focus should be on, "*How do I change enough to get the results I say I want?*"

As a side note, there are some amazing gyms out there too. I love my gym memberships and I've been known to have as many as three memberships at a time, so I can have access to all variety of equipment. Back in the day, Gold's Gym in Kirkland, Washington was wonderful. The focus was on results, camaraderie and mutual interest. That gym location is no longer there, and I believe the owner re-opened a Gold's in Redmond,

Washington....friendly and no sense of the greedy corporate-type of culture. I think the owner's name at that time was John Hamilton.

The majority of new members and personal training clients are *intent* on staying the same, continuing the activity and nutrition lifestyle they have been doing to get fat and unhealthy, yet convincing themselves the gym or trainer (because they paid them) will show them the magic way to live unhealthy, but get the benefits of living a *really fit lifestyle* (perfected-neurosis). Most people show up overfed or underfed, but always malnourished. The cliche 'healthy' or 'balanced' diet is enough if adequate nutrition has been supplied, since the beginning of life, but if you're over weight (body composition of 20% or more) or underweight (lacking lean mass and bone density or showing signs of poor health in your blood chemistry labs), you're already behind nutritionally. Recurrent, nagging injuries or sudden, unexplained injuries also indicate a higher need for nutrition. Without the three-parts of nutrition, the body breaks down.

No amount of exercise or workouts will *put more nutrition in* your body...you can't outrun poor nutrition with any amount of exercise. The only way to get it is to put it in and let nature take over.

Those "last few pounds" are stuck because the body requires nutrition-density (B.N.B.B.s), in order for the body to reverse insulin-resistance and liberate the body fat for energy. Without adequate nutrition-density, energy storage (fat) works only one way (gain fat but can't lose weight). That's why you hear so many people saying they can't get rid of the last five, 10 or 15 pounds of fat...the body is rationing the fat until the nutrition levels go from minimums to a surplus/savings account of the B.N.B.B.s.

To think that exercise alone will make up for poor nutritional habits is irrational, but common among the people who aren't properly fueling their brain enough to function cognitively. Without sensible supplementation of certain dietary supplements, at certain times to make up for gaps in nutrition, you're spinning your wheels insisting you don't understand why you aren't moving. It's the classic case of thinking that not eating correctly for months or years is 'sane', will be made up for with different activity (an exercise program), yet taking supplements is 'extreme'.

(I've never had a client who insisted supplements cost too much, who didn't tell me within the same session about buying coffees, alcohol, chocolate and ice cream, new workout gear, stereo equipment, new sports equipment, etc., etc.). -Values and priorities. If someone values all this other crap over their own nutritional-hygiene, I don't see them as a client.

The reverse is true: allowing *your body* and mind to go with minimum nutrition is extreme, since everything you intend to accomplish is based on a well-nourished brain...purposely withholding the B.N.B.B.s, making excuses, procrastinating getting the B.N.B.B.s etc., is irrational and extreme. Budgeting for your 1) Whole-foods 2) Functional-foods and 3) Certain kinds of dietary supplements at certain times is rational and healthy thinking and personal responsibility. So much so, that I don't work with people if they aren't willing to get these three parts to their nutritional program, in place and follow it consistently on their own.

I'll help people get started for one training cycle, but if they have convinced themselves they know better than me or they simply refuse to prioritize these three nutrition points (skipping the most important parts), I release them to go work with a coach or trainer who will take their money, but, who is neither accountable nor teaches personal responsibility.

Its these clients who skip the three points to a solid nutrition program that keep coming back complaining they didn't get results or that once they got some results in the short-run, they either hit a plateau or the process starts reversing...a mystery!

In the early naive days of my career, I even had clients who wouldn't invest in food, functional-foods or supplements, but insisted their alcohol and pot habit was neither an addiction, a hindrance to progress…another mystery!

How do you know if your program is working?

When I talk about a program working, I'm asking if it: 1) Improves overall health 2) Reduces body fat 3) Improves lean mass 4) Improves strength 5) Improves endurance and stamina 6) Decreases incidence of hereditary conditions and 7) Relieves injury.

How to know for sure your health is improving is to: 1) Before you start your program or now, go to your doctor and have your blood chemistry checked (A1c, blood sugar, cholesterol, triglycerides, blood pressure, etc., etc.). If those markers aren't improving on a quarterly basis, the program (especially the nutritional aspects) are inadequate [no amount of exercise makes up for lack of nutrition-density: B.N.B.B.s].

2) Check your body composition, the first of every month:

The second most important way to know if *the program is working* is you have to check your body composition checked, the first of every month. If you check your body composition less frequently than monthly, you won't know if all the activity is working...are you on track? This is non-negotiable. Without checking your body composition, all activity is random versus being in alignment with your goals and program, designed and based on your goals.

One of the most common (if not THE most common) reasons people complain they aren't getting results or aren't *maintaining the results* they get is because as they progress through their program they aren't updating their program in alignment with their new, updated level of fitness: *doing the same thing over and over without adjusting it as you go results in plateaus in progress.*

If you don't *check your body composition* and adjust it as you go, the workout you're doing this month is outdated...*it was for your level of conditioning from last month!*

Note: BMI is not the same as body composition. Your medical team might want to know BMI because that's how they relate to weight loss vs fat-loss. A person who is at a healthy BMI level, is often way over 20% body fat level (the more over 20% you are, the more likely you are to be vulnerable to diabetes, heart *dis*-ease, high blood pressure, etc., as well as having an imbalanced strength to weight ratio). BMI is not a valid way to measure progress, but your medical team may measure your BMI and tell you, *"You're doing great, keep doing what you're doing."*

Check your body composition, the first of every month, and adjust your daily calories based on the results (more on this later).

3) The third question you want to know is if your calorie requirements are met, to keep getting results:

The outdated idea of "calories-in, calories-out" implies that all you have to do is reduce your calories to lose weight...but what happens when your body requires more calories to stay healthy than you're consuming?

What happens when (as you get more fit, gain lean mass, your calorie requirements INCREASE?). Its backwards right?

You were told to restrict calories, but at a certain point (about 90 days) you've reduced your calories as much as you can, but now you're gaining weight back...how does that make sense?

HINT: As you *get more fit*, (from the exercise), you gain lean mass as you're simultaneously burning fat. As you *gain lean mass*, even though you *appear* and feel *smaller* and your clothes are fit better, YOUR CALORIC REQUIREMENTS INCREASE.

That means that (even though counter-intuitively), as you get more fit, your calorie requirements increase (to a point). If you don't adjust your calories the first of the month, based on your new, current fitness level (for the previous month) the metabolism slows, plateaus and even begins to reverse...*without enough calories the body begins rationing and adding back more fat.*

Adding more exercise (duration, intensity and/or frequency) only compounds the problem...meaning the more exercise you do while consuming too few calories the problem becomes worse. If you slip into this mode of doing more and consuming too few calories, you've essentially put yourself back into beginner mode...*malnourished and over trained.* **No amount of exercise will make up for inadequate nutrition/calories...you can't outrun poor nutrition with any amount of exercise.**

So, use an online calorie calculator. The one I have successfully used since 2006 is below:

http://www.dietitian.com/calcbody.php

When you get to this website, you'll notice that in order to accurately establish your current calorie requirements you have to know your body composition (how much fat you have and how much lean mass you have). Without those numbers, calories are guessed but without consideration for your current fitness level.

See the pattern? The first of the month, recheck your: 1) Body composition 2) Your calorie requirements and 3) Your resting and target heart rates. Without doing these calculations the first of each month, you'll likely lose lean mass and gain body fat as your workouts continue.

Let's get into the specific of your workouts.

Chapter Eight

Designing An Exercise Program;
Resistance-Training

Did you know there was a study at Cleveland State University that showed that people who exercise, at least three times per week, earn ten-percent more than those who don't? In my personal training business, I've seen this over and over. Often, people who have never exercised consistently, begin to notice their career and lifestyle improving, in relation to the consistency with which they apply nutrition and exercise. Out of seemingly nowhere, the more consistent they are with their habits, the more opportunities come their way.

When designing an exercise program, there's a few things you have to consider. First and foremost is safety. If your program isn't designed with safety in mind, you'll likely get hurt. Where this often shows up as when people either begin exercising for the first time, or they have had some time off or they're simply progressing too quickly, for where their fitness level is today. People often think that because they started a program they can start adding in all kinds of exercise, which leads to injury.

To be safe, you have to consider where your perceptions of what exercise program you're considering are. In other words, a most common mistake is to know what you want your body to look and perform like, but decide on a program that has no way of producing the *results you* say you *want.* One of the dichotomies we have as humans is the ability to say we want one thing, but insist we're going to do action that gets the opposite of what we say we want...we call it freedom, anonymity or independence...then we complain we didn't get what we wanted!

The basis of how I train people is whole-body, resistance-training also known as weight-training. The reason being that the health and performance benefits are so broad and wide ranging that whole books are written on all the benefits of resistance-training.

For the sake of burning fat, gaining strength, gaining lean mass and improving endurance as well as improving all those nasty health conditions we are told are normal and average, resistance-training can't be beat. In addition, resistance-training done properly, acts as a barometer of weak links, in the body. Ideally, the conscientious athlete focuses on strengthening the weak links *first*, rather than working what is already strong and neglecting the weak links. Weak links can be areas of restriction or maladaptive shortening, which indicates unconscious holding patterns and groups of muscles which may be working against each other and contributes to low-back pain, neck pain and knee pain. These can show up as injuries in the major muscle groups such as hamstrings, glutes and the hip areas. More common than not, the problem with the major muscle is the superficial symptom of weaker dysfunction, in areas of the body that seem unrelated.

Frequency:

Specifically, I'm talking about three sessions, per week, with a day of rest in between, each resistance-training session lasting 50-60 minutes in duration.

This is a full body workout, where over the course of a week or two, you'll work up to three sets, of each exercise, per body part.

Always begin your resistance-training, with a brief warm up, say five to ten minutes on a stationary-bike, where you get the bigger muscle groups and the cardiovascular-system warmed up.

The first time you do this workout, you'll do one set each exercise, then see how you' feel in the two days after the workout. If you're not sore at all, do two sets the following workout. If you are sore after doing two sets, you'll stick with two sets until you are no longer sore in the couple days following that workout. If you're not sore two days after your workout, you'll progress to three sets per body part during the next workout and maintain three sets per body part for each workout after that.

It's important to aim for 50 minutes of resistance-training, but say you're at a gym and have to wait on a machine or rested more for some reason, you can top off the workout at 60 minutes. Whatever you didn't complete within this 50-60 minutes, you skip and begin with those exercises during your next workout (this builds in a kind of 'rollover recovery factor'). Especially for beginners or people *getting back on track* it's important to emphasize recovery, so there's no practical reason to do more than an hour of resistance-training, three-times, per week. If you have more time to exercise you would want to incorporate other categories of exercises, that I'll talk about later. There is the phenomena you have to watch out for, where people think more is better (time/duration) or working too hard for their current level of fitness/conditioning (intensity). That's part of the reason I teach the idea of *leaving some gas in the tank*...if you do so, not only are you going to be recovering better and creating resistance to injury and illness you'll feel a lot better and come into each workout/training session stronger and more fresh.

This is a whole-body workout, meaning one exercise per body part, working up to three sets, per exercise. Be present with the task at hand, meaning focus on the muscle group you're working at the time. For people who tend to get hurt frequently, this points to lack of being present (having awareness of self) in their body (focusing on the past or the future rather than being completely present). As you raise the weight (the heavy part of the exercise/contraction phase/concentric) exhale. As you lower the weight (the weight pulling you down/relaxation phase/eccentric) you exhale every repetition. The breathing will help keep you present, help generate proper power, prevent and alleviate improper tension as well as make you strong but relaxed.

Before each set, use all your senses to *imagine* you have just successfully completed the next set, before you begin it. See yourself having *completed* the reps, feel the accomplishment. This is multi-purpose, including preparing your body for the upcoming exercise, but it carries over to all areas of success; mastering *rehearsal of success*. Once you have it clear that you have already accomplished the lift/set, do the actual set. You can apply this to all athletic/fitness activity including the nutritional aspects which tend to have a high emotional-resistance threshold (use it to break old habits and create new ones). Whether running, cycling, swimming or whatever, visualize the success ahead of time. Just make sure you include the *feelings* that *you have just completed it successfully* and the feelings that go with *success*. Without emotionally 'charging' visualization, just 'seeing' it isn't as potent or thorough. Including the emotions of success is how the brain embodies what it is you intend to do. Just like anything, if you don't know how to do this, practice it. Develop it, in yourself.

In between each set, you *focus on relaxing* the body via [relaxation stretching]. There's a few types of stretching, but during these workouts your intent is to relax and slightly lengthen the muscle you just worked, by deeply breathing and essentially placing the muscle into a mildly elongated position, but without the force most people think of when they hear the word 'stretching'.

Again, the idea is to relax the muscle (allow it to lengthen) not force it into a stretch that causes it to cramp or contract or get strained, which leads to chronic injury. A common theme in my style of personal training is that the body will improve anyway (regardless of the type of training) if you're consistent so pushing or forcing the body versus giving hints and allowing the body to improve only sets you up for injury, setbacks and time off from hasty choices.

I've found that if you *focus on a relaxation*-lengthening of each muscle, between sets for 30 seconds, on each side (left and right) while breathing and thinking "relax" that within about seven seconds, you'll feel the muscle let go out of the contracted state...but you sustain that length for 30 seconds. Each workout the *relaxation* response naturally increases. Not only does this help the muscles physically relax, it trains the body (at the hormone and nervous system levels) to expect a *relaxation* phase (parasympathetic response) following any stress phase (sympathetic response). Most people adapt to daily stress by storing stress in their body, which simply makes you more and more stressed out as time goes on.

Preventing overtraining:

Also known as the General Adaptation Syndrome (G.A.S.), people think that as long as they can 'keep going' the stress isn't hurting or affecting them. But inside the body the stress is affecting them and building up, which has a breaking down effect on the organs and systems of the body. So, by taking the minute or more to stretch between sets you're actually training your body to switch back from a stress response to a relaxation response, outside your awareness...*a healthy, unconscious habit.*

People who don't stretch between sets generally end up with tight, maladapted muscles which creates imbalances on the joints and in turn are really setting themselves up for serious injury. The muscles also recover from each set faster, by stretching, which means you'll feel better and more ready, for your next set.

A lot of my clients have told me how tired they used to be after workouts prior to training with me, but this style of relaxing between sets leads to feeling more energized and relaxed and mentally clear following the resistance-training than before. In other words, when done properly, your energy will be higher after your workouts than before, due to releasing tension and stimulating the nervous and hormone systems versus beating them up.

In the beginning phases, I prefer my clients use flat plate loaded machines like you see at any modern gym. *Nautilus* and *Life Fitness* are great examples, but any brand will do, as long as the seat and settings for limb placement are adjustable to fit you and the proper placement of your joints. My primary reasons for this is that we want to load the resistance on your muscles and tendons, not your joints and ligaments. Modern, plate loaded machines do this wonderfully. I've had clients who want to train at home and that's your choice point...a place where you can remove, alter or change the program before you even get started, but you'll miss out on a lot of the key benefits...you simply won't get as good of results.

If you have zero experience with resistance-training (weight lifting) your focus will be on doing three sets of each exercise.

The first set you'll set the weight so that (with proper form and safety) you can do no more than 10 repetitions and then get up and do the stretching for relaxation for each muscle you work. You should *gently* lengthen the muscle while *breathing* for at least one-minute (30 seconds each side). After stretching and while recovering from the set, visualize completing the next set as described earlier.

If you and a friend are training together, you'll have more rest time while they are doing their sets.

Once you have worked up to two sets per exercise, the second set you'll rest the weight, so you can only do eight reps for that set, meaning the weight is heavy enough that eight is the most you can do and maintain good, safe form. Then you go into your stretching for *relaxation* again between every set.

What I want you to do in *linger in the relaxation* stretching phase, between sets. Allow the body to relax. Ultimately, your strength is going to be higher and you'll make better progress by resting between sets anyway (your strength will be higher by resting 1-3 minutes between each set). One of the common mistakes people make is disregarding that the body has to rest between sets, during weight training, so they go too fast, rest too little and miss a lot of the benefits of the workout itself. As you progress, your strength will increase *pretty quickly,* if your nutrition is dialed-in, so you'll need more rest *to recover* from heavier weights (one to three minutes between each set).

If you don't feel like you can do the relax-stretching and rest a little between sets, then that has to do with *calming* your mind and emotions down; getting present. A side-affect of being distracted, anxious, disassociated and so forth is the inability to stay focused and complete tasks. Being fit is a result, of being present in the body, at the moment. Being present is one of the qualities you'll want to cultivate so that the time you invest during your workouts is efficient.

Once you have worked up to your third set, you'll set the weight so you can do no more than six, quality, full range of motion repetitions for the third set.

Its common in the beginning to underestimate your strength and that's no big deal, meaning maybe the first set you set the weight where you were last workout, but you easily did 12 reps instead of fatiguing at 10 reps, simply make a note of it, that means you gained strength during your rest days since your last workout. Maybe your third set you're *aiming* for six reps and you could do four reps. That's not a big deal either, just make a note that you overestimated your strength. Most likely during your next workout you'll easily do six reps with the same weight! (adaptation). By aiming for six, but only making it to four, will stimulate strength anyway. I just want to you aim for six reps on your third set, so you aren't going so heavy that your risk poor form and injury, in order to move the weight...you're going to get stronger with time anyway! And you don't want to go so light that you do eight or ten reps in your third set.

By doing this 10,8,6 rep range you'll be stimulating strength, lean mass, endurance and at the same time building up the conditioning of your ligaments and tendons without going so heavy you hurt yourself. It takes a good six to eight-weeks to go through the basis of making the connective tissues (tissue other than muscle) able to handle exercise and to keep the joints safe. You don't want your muscles to get stronger faster than what the tendons and ligaments can handle, Secondly, by adhering to this rep range you'll find what areas are weak or need more improvement, without placing so much stress that the area gets hurt and then prevents you from working out at all.

Ideally, you want to focus on *improving* the weakest areas first and foremost during each workout. Most people focus on working the areas they are already stronger in then being surprised when their muscular system gets imbalanced and end up with shoulder, hip and/or back injuries (sign of underlying weak links and the stronger muscles being stronger, yet dangerously shortened, thereby placing strange stress on the joints that has to be compensated for elsewhere in the body). The majority of people ignore the weak links because they aren't as *fun* to train in the beginning and then wonder why they got injured!

If you have been working out for at least eight-weeks already, doing resistance-training (weight-training) for at least eight-weeks, then the principles are the same, but you'll do a rep range of 12,10,8,6 (four sets total for each exercise).

The reason for this rep range, is to *allow* a little more warm up, *preparing* for the heavier fourth set, and allow for more recovery during the sets, since you've gotten stronger during the first eight-weeks. 12 reps tend to be where the most muscle is stimulated, but if you do 12 reps all the time you won't develop any significant strength. So, the six reps on the last set stimulates strength so that as you progress you're doing more weight in the 12 rep range in later workouts. You'll still utilize the 'rollover *recovery* process' meaning what you don't get done within 50-60 minutes is what you begin your workout with the following workout. There's no benefit to doing this 12,10,6 rep range if you haven't spent at least eight-weeks doing the 10,8,6 rep range so don't jump ahead thinking you'll get faster results, just the opposite. It's just that you'll have an idea of what your workouts will look like in weeks eight through fourteen or sixteen.

The 10,8,6 rep cycle places emphasis on (intensity/strength) while the 12,10,6 places more on total (volume/amount) of exercise, giving your body a break from eight-weeks of pushing for heavier weight each workout, which you can't do indefinitely without overtraining and getting hurt or at least burned out, while the third set of six reps permits maintenance of the strength you developed, within the first eight-week cycle.

Time to burn some fat.

Chapter Nine

Designing An Exercise Program;
Fat-Burning Cardio

One of the interesting phenomena seasoned trainers notice, with their clients who insist they are committed, is that they want to "hurry-up-and-get-going" but, then won't stick to the program (the "hurry-up-and-procrastinate" behavior).

In the big picture, how I suggest *looking* at your routine is to *make nutrition* (whole-foods, functional-foods *and* certain supplements at certain times), the highest and *most important priority*, followed by resistance-training (which builds lean mass and is the basis of a consistent metabolism) followed by fat-burning, cardiovascular-training to burn off the excess fat (anything more than 20% body composition for non-athletes; anything more than 10%-15%, for athletic types).

By *prioritizing* in *this* order (nutrition, resistance-training, cardio) you'll get better results than most people who are putting in the same amounts of time and energy and money but, prioritized differently.

Nutrition (whole-foods, functional-foods and certain kinds of dietary supplements at certain times), provides what your *body* needs to carry out the *signals* which resistance-training and fat-burning cardio are supposed to provide. Without these three components the efforts you put into your workouts won't produce full results...in other words, you'll put the same amount or even more time and energy into your workouts, but your body won't respond fully since the *body requires nutrition-density* provided in consistent quality, quantity and timing in order to respond to the training itself. That's not to say you won't *get* some *results* (or get results in the first months) you simply won't get the level you would once you dial-in the three components I refer to throughout this book. You'll begin getting full results the day you make sure you're getting all three parts of nutrition.

More often than not, the people who are complaining they aren't getting any results from their workouts, or *results* are slow, inconsistent or they're even gaining fat and losing lean mass are disregarding and dismissing the three nutritional components. I hope the importance of this is clear and adhered to.

Fat-burning cardio:

In order to structure your cardio-sessions to really *get* your body to tap into that bodyfat and/or the stubborn areas of your body, you want to get very specific and *consistent* with 'how' you do your cardio. You want the majority of your time doing cardio-specific training (as opposed to resistance-training) to be in what 'seems' like a lower intensity range of exertion...a range that to the novice seems too easy to do any good (another place where the "hurry up and procrastinate" pattern rears its head: *having procrastinated to get started on a professionally designed program, only to not stick with a program, imagining it isn't intense enough to make up for all the procrastinating, thereby sabotaging the magic of consistently applying a properly designed program*).

More often than not, people think 'more is better' and that includes higher-intensity, cardio-sessions that we mistake for activity which will give faster results...*more is better, right?* Like I've said before, much of the exercise and activity we think we see other people *getting results* from, whether online, in the gym or where ever don't provide consistent, measurable results, nor are they sustainable. In other words, high-intensity training provides some change in the short-run (or is used to introduce variety into a consistent program) but, often ultimately leads to over-training, injury, burn out and more procrastination, in the form of exercise avoidance, when done too often.

Remember how I said the first of each month you have to check your resting heart rate (RHR), body composition (body fat % compared to lean mass) and adjust your calorie consumption? Generally, the high-intensity type cardio programs focus on activity, but fail miserably at training the body to burn excess body fat for energy. In other words, the person might be jumping around doing all kinds of crazy moves and breathing like crazy, sweating all over the place, but when you check their body fat level, the first of the month they often have lost lean mass and gained fat. It's not uncommon at all for a person doing one of the infomercial-type workouts to have what they call 'trouble spots' like the hips, abs or arms that they can't seem to rid the fat of and insist they are doing everything right but can't lose the last "15 pounds"...the reason being they are active, exerting themselves, but not training the body to burn fat for energy...*simply doing entertaining or random activity*...a symptom of not investing energy in proper program design.

If your three nutrition components are dialed-in and your resistance-training and cardio is dialed-in, your metabolism is running efficiently enough that you literally are burning fat, while sleeping.

With that in mind, it's really important to learn what fat-burning cardio means, how to set it up for yourself and then stick to it and adjust it as you go (monthly) as you become more fit (noted by the decrease in your resting heart rate).

What it is:

Remember there's essentially three types of cardio-training. Some burns fat, some does cardiovascular conditioning so the heart functions better and some is designed for maximum output, during high-intensity athletics like long distance Nordic skiing, cycling and running.

All three types have some things in common (they all improve function and health *to an extent*) but, fat-burning cardio is sustainable/maintainable, has a very low likelihood of injury and is really efficient at *getting* the body to tap into the most stubborn fat reserves (note: trouble spots, cellulite, etc., are symptoms of insulin-resistance , meaning the body stores fat but doesn't use it for energy, so it accumulates even though exercise is being done), which stay in place or even *expand* if exercise intensity isn't correlated with your current fitness level and age adjusted training level (Karvonen Method: as described, shortly here).

How much?

Twenty-minutes, three times a week (with a day in between each session for rest) following the fifty-minute, resistance-training sessions is where to *start*. Yes, make sure you perform it *after* the resistance-training.

Set yourself up for success:

Part of what sets this kind of cardio apart is that you'll be doing the exercise, within your actual fitness level, versus some idea you came up with randomly or by watching someone else...it's based on your fitness level, which is measured by your personal resting heart rate (RHR) and your, age not by simply doing the most intense workout you're capable of.

Critical:

In order to do fat-burning cardio effectively, you'll *remind yourself* that the first of the month, first thing in the morning when you wake up, before you even sit up, check your heart rate/pulse. Measure it for one-minute, wait one-minute and then take it again (this is your RHR, which tells us how fit you are and leads to accurately setting up your fat-burning cardio, for your specific body). Put it on your appointment calendar.

This number, your pulse/RHR is valid for one month. Regardless what day you first check your RHR, recheck it on the first of the month and continue to do so, indefinitely. Checking your RHR the first of each month is to develop the habit so you know for sure you're in your particular training-zone for burning fat (most people skip this step, train randomly and insist they can't burn fat/"*...have tried everything*"/that "*...it isn't working*".).

If you don't check your RHR (leaving too much to chance), you'll likely be training too intensely or not intensely enough to target the fat, thereby losing lean mass (healthy tissue) and continuing to gain fat even though you're exercising wasting time, energy and resources.

What day do you check your RHR? *The first of each month.* **Which day?** *The first of each month.* **Which day?** *The first of each month.*

Karvonen Method for your fat-burning target heart rate zone:

Once you know where your resting heart rate is (how many heart beats per minute) you'll use these numbers to find out the 60%-70% of your maximum training zone (60%-70% is where you'll invest a majority of your time for fat-burning cardio).

To figure out your own cardio zone each month, you'll do this:

220 minus your age minus RHR x 60% + RHR = the minimum of your training zone.

and also:

220 minus your age minus- RHR x 70% + RHR = the maximum of your training zone.

For example:

Because graphics and photos are so limited, you can request my article that details this in detail by emailing me requesting *The Fat-burning Cardio Special Report.*

The big picture:

For fat-burning cardio, part of the time (one-minute at a time) is spent above the 60%-70% THR, of your maximum training zone (and no more than one-minute at a time), while the alternating minutes you'll be in the lower intensity of 60%-70% to allow your heart rate to return to 60%-70% of your max heart rate.

How long you stay at the lower zone (60%-70%) depends on how long it takes for your heart rate to lower/return after you reach the 60%-70% of your maximum training zone. The more fit you are cardiovascular wise, the faster your heart rate will return to 60%-70%. Once your heart rate lowers to 60%-70%, for one-minute then you raise the intensity back up, enough that your heart goes above the 60%-70% of your maximum training zone, for one-minute once again.

Note: On the higher levels, above 60%-70%, as soon as one-minute passes, *immediately* return to the lower training zone (not waiting to do so or tapering gradually; *immediate*).

The time (between) each of your 60%-70% of your maximum training zones is however long it takes to allow your heart rate to return back to 60%-70% of your maximum training zone.

In the beginning (if you're out of shape) it might take three minutes to return to 60%-70% of your maximum heart rate, after raising the level above 60%-70%.

By alternating in and out of your 60%-70% of your maximum training zone you're training at an intensity that taps into the body fat for energy but effectively preserves the energy stores that make up lean mass (everything besides the body fat/healthy tissue).

In the first month, I suggest these cardio-sessions are 20 minutes in length, following your resistance-training session.

How?

I always get the questions like, *"Can't I just go for a walk?"* or *"Can't I just go out and jog?"*

Truthfully, what people need to do is use some sort of stationary exercise machine that allows choices in the programming, but set the machine to "manual". Ideally, this is a stationary bike. Remember, the idea is to learn how to optimally get your metabolism into a fat-burning zone. If you can't control all the variables from the beginning, then there's too many variables to stabilize our heart rate within the 60%-70% and to differentiate how to get your heart rate to lower than this immediately at the one-minute mark, for each spike in resistance/intensity above your 60%-70%.

If you already have adequate experience tracking your heart rate (preferably with some sort of electronic device) then it doesn't matter how you go about the ups and downs within the cardio session, but for most people trying to maintain proper intensity and walking outside or jogging is too much to pay attention to get your program dialed-in, within nine workouts. Without standardizing your workout on a stationary bike, there's too many variables to get a hold on what to do and what not to do. What happens is people either can't get their heart rate high enough (on time) or they aren't in good enough shape to get their heart rate high enough to burn fat but walking or doing something outdoors. The idea is to reduce all the variables and distractions and focus on conditioning your metabolism/rate of fat-burning.

Time and time again clients ask if they can't just go outdoors and *"...try it without a boring machine,"* only to not follow through. Today I more or less interpret this kind of questions as within the "hurry up and procrastinate" realm, where the client is making excuses, picking the program apart before they start it and asking for permission to not follow through and then claim the program doesn't work.

Cardio, if viewed in one light can be thought of as boring...many people, even professional athletes can think of it this way. It can be tedious in a sense. But the people who get amazing results with their fitness program and workouts are the ones that make the program work for them. Meaning they have music, watch movies, listen to audio books, etc., during their cardio-sessions to MAKE the cardio enjoyable. The people who get amazing results are the ones who do the work regardless of their opinion of the work during the process. You have to make the process *enjoyable,* in your own mind, in your own way.

If this is the first time you've ever done a program like this, then you have to stay focused on the *results* and the payoff you'll get over the coming months. You have to create and *have faith* it works when you do it consistently and correctly and you stick to it.

For me, I simply focus on the payoff I get from workout-to-workout and *enjoy* pushing myself as well as learning about how my body responds to exercise and that's enough to get through it. I usually have music and TV going. Studies have shown that listening to music while exercising relives boredom, increases tolerance to exercise, distracts from work and exertion and people tend to simply do better by listening to upbeat *music,* it's that simple.

In the first one to nine workouts, when you're *learning* how to set the bike up for yourself, you might be working at too low of intensity and not get to your 60%-70% target heart rate (THR) and that's ok. The idea is to *learn something in each workout.* Each workout you'll raise or tweak the intensity a bit, so you get the bike set where you are closer to your zone. If you don't have your training set, within three weeks (9 workouts) then something is off, and you'll want to ask me for help.

Additionally, how you standardize your intensity is most stationary bikes have a number that shows how fast you are pedaling. You want to be doing about 55-60 revolutions per minute, regardless what level of intensity you're at. Sometimes this is shown as speed "10-11" on the electronic screen. My ProForm bike I have, at home, shows a little differently so it's in the speed of 10-11. The idea is to get used to each pedal making a full revolution each second. If your particular bike has a different way to measure, ask me for help.

20-minute example for beginner:

The idea is to start the session low intensity and gradually increase without going above your sixty to seventy percent training zone during the base level, in intensity that you set yourself. The two minutes can be a warm up, but you'll be doing this after your resistance-training, so you'll be pretty warmed up already.

It's more important to do twenty minutes correctly than to do extended or longer sessions with random intensity, too much intensity or too little intensity.

Notice that in the following example, each increment the intensity is manually changed, in order to ultimately find where you need to be, this month for your 60%-70% of your maximum heart rate. Meaning, in the beginning you might not know where to set the resistance, so it will take some experimenting (learn something every workout). But, you don't have to know it all, simply experiment so in alternating minutes you're in your 60%-70% of your maximum heart rate, and then raise the intensity so you're above 60%-70% of your maximum heart rate, until your heart rate returns for one-minute, followed by decreasing the intensity/resistance to 60%-70% of your maximum heart rate (THR).

In the following example, manual level 2 represents where a person with very little experience or conditioning lowers the intensity to in order to get their heart rate within 60%-70% of their maximum heart rate (THR) and that's why its repeated through the workout.

As the weeks pass (and as your conditioning improves) the level 2 will become a 3 and then a 4 and so on (again, the importance of checking your RHR the first of the month, to see how your conditioning has improved:

Minutes 1-2: manual level 2; heart rate 60%-70% (THR)

Minute 2-3: manual level 3; above THR

Minute 3-4: manual level 2; heart rate 60%-70% (THR)

Minute 4-5: manual level 3; above THR

Minute 5-6: manual level 2; heart rate 60%-70% (THR)

Minute 6-7: manual level 4; above THR

Minute 7-8: manual level 2; heart rate 60%-70% (THR)

Minute 8-9: manual level 5; above THR

Minute 9-10: manual level 2; heart rate 60%-70% (THR)

Minute 10-11: manual level 6; above THR

Minute 11-12: manual level 2; heart rate 60%-70% (THR)

Minute 12-13: manual level 6; above THR

Minute 13-14: manual level 2; heart rate 60%-70% (THR)

Minute 14-15: manual level 7; above THR

Minute 15-16: manual level 2; heart rate 60%-70% (THR)

Minute 16-17: manual level 7; above THR

Minute 18-20: manual level 2; heart rate 60%-70% (THR)

(cool down)

Note that whatever level or however low the intensity level is (base level), in order to allow your heart rate to return to 60%-70% (THR) is fine and doesn't matter, it's the fact that you allow the heart rate to lower to 60%-70% (THR) of your maximum heart rate, rather than staying in the higher intensity/resistance, for more than one-minute.

The level that puts you within your zone isn't going to be the same for anyone else and that's the point. Its based on your current fitness kevel/resting heart rate (RHR)

In the beginning sessions, you won't know how your target 60%-70% correlates with the intensity that you set the bike at and that's ok, no one expects you to know that.

It takes a little back and forth *experimenting*, but it's more important in the first three weeks/9 workouts to train at less than your target heart rate than to go too fast or too intense and go above your training zone...again, avoid the 'hurry up and procrastinate' mindset and think long-term with little improvements/refinements, each workout. If you're doing any cardio at all and increasing the intensity levels at all, you'll be getting more fit, and improving anyway. Going too fast (doing too much intensity too quickly) is a different kind of cheating that will bite you. Lower intensity is better, considering you're doing this fat-burning cardio, after your resistance-training sessions.

Even though, in this example, the person started at level two for the first one to three minutes, as the weeks go by and your fitness level improves, the "base" or starting level (the lower level used to return to 60%-70% (THR) will also increase, meaning your fitness will improve so your minimums will increase also, meaning you'll notice your heart rate below your target zone as your base level increases (improved cardiovascular fitness).

The point of saying you figured out (within three weeks or nine workouts) is to allow for people who are adjusting their workouts themselves that they don't have to do it perfectly from the beginning, just make consistent improvements, which add up, but to set a time limit to make sure you're paying enough attention to get it dialed-in, within a reasonable time frame.

If you decide to participate in athletic events later (once you get your body fat composition 20% or less), then you would alternate fat-burning cardio-sessions with cardiovascular training sessions. But, if you really think it through, as you continue on with fat-burning cardio, your fitness improves and so the levels you train at, increases as the weeks go by and ultimately you're doing cardiovascular training anyway...it's just that its within your fitness thresh hold and you're not having any of the side-effects of over training or training too intensely to be sustainable.

This example is for twenty minutes as a good rule of thumb for consistent/sustainable results. Ultimately, *you can* do longer sessions as long as you stick to the same structure. You could potentially do 30-minute sessions, following your resistance-training if you wanted or do two 20 minute sessions (one immediately following your resistance-training) as long as you stick to the structure described, but you would also have to *adjust* your calorie intake (increase) or you'll end up likely getting in a caloric deficit and end up losing lean mass and gaining fat in the long run.

Note: It's more important to get your fat-burning cardio dialed-in (so you know where and how to access your target heart rate is) than to do longer or more frequent sessions (quality vs quantity).

Novice trainers and clients often mistake this kind of fat-burning cardio as 'interval' training, which this is not. Interval training has different effects and tends to push the heart rate too high to preserve lean mass (burns calories but compromises lean mass in the process). So, if you do interval training and say that's what I showed you, you'll likely end up complaining it didn't work. This is not interval training...this works better, faster and is more sustainable in the long run since it's based on your current fitness level and age (RHR/Karvonen method) as opposed to what is known as perceived exertion level and is more subjective than objective.

This particular style permits you to more *easily* track your progress and in turn provides you the information so that you reduce the likelihood of having plateaus/sticking points, as well as makes it so *you know* how to change and what to change as you progress through the months instead of hitting a plateau and not knowing what needs to change to continue *making progress!*

Now, let's cover how to know how well your program is working.

Chapter Ten

How To Measure Your Body Composition

Q: Do you remember when to check your body composition?

A: *The first of each month.*

There are many ways and devices to measure body composition (how much fat compared to lean mass you have). *Your first goal is to reach 20% or less body fat.*

Regardless of which device you use whether it is a manual, hand-held caliper or a handheld electronic device or a huge, clinical or academic device you sit in or lie down in water, *you want* to use the same device and procedure, the first of each month.

The reason being is that there is significant difference between each device (10% or more) even if you measure within minutes, with each device. I prefer the handheld calipers for their overall simplicity and because I've used them for decades and know how *to use them correctly,* but they do require a second person to read the numbers, on the places on the back of the body you can't reach yourself.

Note: Even though each body composition device varies as much as 10%, the main thing you're monitoring for is a trend of improvement (less fat and more lean mass) or a trend of regression (loss of lean mass and gain of fat).

These kind of results show how well the previous four weeks of nutrition, resistance and cardio are dialed-in for your body. Without checking, all activity is random, unpredictable and leaves people disappointed...it doesn't happen by accident!

There's about eight variations that will show up when you check your body composition, so in the next chapter I tell you what each variation means so *you* know what to *change* in your program...nothing is left to chance or question here.

Some of the electronic, handheld devices will give a reading if they are held at heart level in front of you with straight arms, a lower reading if your arms are below heart level and a higher reading if your arms are higher than heart level. So, you have to make sure you follow manufacturer guidelines accurately, so you know for sure whether you made improvements or regressed (gain body fat and/or lost lean mass), since your last check in.

At one gym I trained at they had an electronic handheld body comp device and I would watch the trainers taking body composition on their clients without reading the instructions. Its subtle, but some trainers would have the client hold the device in front and above them, when they started training and as they progressed, progressively lower their hands which caused a lower reading. The clients never knew the difference, but to them all they saw was the body composition numbers going down with time, which even if their body weight didn't change it would imply they were gaining lean mass and getting leaner. Yes...if someone started training with me I told them. But I was busy six to eight hours a day with my own clients...it's the nature of the gym business and that's why I'm telling you here...if it's a handheld device where both hands are holding it and your arms are out in front of you, make sure your hands are level with your heart.

If someone helps you do the body composition check (say with the calipers) make sure the same person helps you each time (consistent use is key). Many trainers don't know how to use them correctly to begin with. Calipers also come with an instruction booklet.

I use the *Slim Guide Skin Fold Caliper with booklet* which is available from Amazon for about twenty-bucks. I also have a body composition scale I bought on Amazon, for about thirty-bucks, which also measures BMI, hydration level, bone density and body weight.

The key is to get whatever one you'll consistently use. The whole idea is to keep track of what changes occur from the three points of a complete nutrition program: (1) Whole-foods 2) Functional-foods and 3) Certain supplements at certain times and your 4) Resistance-training and 5) Fat-burning cardio.

If you don't track your body composition, the first of each month, then you won't know if your program is working (you'll be investing time, energy and resources) and wondering why you aren't getting consistent results. Imagine working a program for two months, only to find out you gained fat and lost lean mass! Its more common than not. Checking body-composition, the first of each month is non-negotiable.

The first of each month you check your body composition. There are about 8 variations of what you might see.

Chapter Eleven

Understanding What The
Body Composition Numbers Mean,
And What To Do About It.

The first of each month, *when you check* your resting heart rate (RHR), reset your target heart rate (THR), based on you RHR, and recalculate your caloric requirements you'll also check your body composition (percentage of body fat, compared to lean mass).

There are about eight variations of the numbers that if you don't notice at first, down the road you will, since caloric estimations and estimations of how much *exercise you need* to reach and maintain your goal(s) are just that...best, professional guesses on available information. You really don't know how good your estimation were, until after applying it for a month, you recheck your numbers. The more consistent you are, month-after-month, the better and more dialed-in your guesses are (getting to know your body/developing instincts) (correct actions combined with accurate measurements, leads to instincts).

So, for the sake of simplicity we'll use the number 100 pounds of bodyweight here. Bodyweight by itself doesn't tell us if we improved our fitness level by increasing/decreasing body fat, nor improved or regressed in lean mass. If we only weighed ourselves on the scale it wouldn't tell how much of our weight is healthy or unhealthy...so we measure body composition (percentage of body fat compared to lean mass).

So, on day one/month one this fictional person "Bob" weighs 100 pounds for this fictional, but common example, we'll say Bob has 30% body fat (10% more than the first goal of 20%) and 20% lean mass.

Each 1% of body fat is approximately 2 pounds of fat, in the beginning of a program, for someone above 20% bodyfat. The more over 20% the more you're getting into the danger zone for the *de*-generative *dis*-eases like diabetes, heart *dis*-ease, injuries, etc. So, your first goal is to get to 20% body fat.

Example #1: Lost Lean Mass:

So, for this fictional account, thirty-days has passed/one month. The first-of-the-month rolls around and Bob measures his body composition for the second time, to see how he did the first month.

Bob's numbers show that his body fat stayed the same, but he lost some lean mass

30% body fat (same)/15% lean mass(lost)/[a 5% decrease in lean mass].

Losing lean mass is a sign of either eating too few calories or doing too intense cardio for Bob's current fitness level (with the three resistance-workouts and three fat-burning cardio-sessions, the body was tapping into the lean mass and preserving the body fat). Assuming Bob followed the guidelines accurately for checking his RHR and having a cardio base level of 60% -70% we have to estimate his calorie consumption was too low, since low intensity cardio wouldn't use muscle/lean mass for energy...his overall activity level needs more calories. If he didn't stick to the fat-burning cardio guidelines, then we wouldn't know with much certainty which factor caused the loss of lean mass. In this case, the loss of lean mass points to too few calories.

If the same thing happens two months in a row, then that would suggest Bob saying he is doing one thing as suggested, but doing something entirely different...he needs supervision since he lacks enough awareness to even follow through on the guidelines.

So, for example #1 Bob maintained his fat but lost lean mass, so he needs to increase his calories by 300-500, on each day he exercises. If it's truly a caloric issue, the second month would show an increase in lean mass (at least to where he started from) and likely a decrease in fat mass (burning fat requires eating enough calories).

Example #2: Maintained Fat & Gained Lean Mass:

As a follow up to Example #1, this is where Bob wants to be, at least at first.

A lot of people are overly-concerned, with burning fat, to the point that they subconsciously begin to starve themselves by "forgetting" to eat whole-foods, functional-foods or skipping certain kinds of supplements at certain times (making excuses). Most of the population thinks they can out-smart Mother Nature and make "weight" loss happen faster by either forgetting to eat or actively withholding food and nutrition to make the exercise work faster. Common yes, but so is losing some weight fast and then hitting a plateau and gaining even more weight back than in the beginning.

So in month two, Bob had gained some "weight". If you looked at the scale (but ignored body composition) you might even see a decrease in body 'weight" but in a negative way, since the scale doesn't tell you if you lost healthy lean mass (bad thing) or lost unhealthy body fat (good thing).

Bob's body fat remained the same (30%) [which is fine because he's now way more fit and has a foundation of lifelong fitness to build on] and his lean mass had recovered and gained some going from 20% in the beginning to 15% during the first month to 25% during the second month...the direction you want to go in.

Part of the possible reason why (in this example Bob's body fat didn't change) is because he is still learning/dialing-in his cardio (which can take up the three weeks/he hasn't been consistent enough with his 60%-70% target heart rate range to burn fat and retain lean mass/doesn't have a track record of success to build on). If someone actually has a trainer right there with them, their cardio should be dialed-in within three sessions (if the trainer knows what they're doing). Without a trainer there, we have to assume it might take a little longer to adjust and interpret the numbers and what's going on in the body.

In reality, if Bob simply followed the guidelines for the three parts of nutrition, resistance and cardio to a "T" he would have likely lost 12-20 pounds of fat the first month and gained at least ten pounds of lean mass. The point is to learn how to adjust based on body composition numbers until you get to your optimal fitness level from then on.

Example #3: Lost Lean Mass & Gained or Maintained Fat:

Unfortunately, Bob was exercising his right to 'hurry-up and procrastinate' and Bob didn't check any of his numbers, in month one (RHR, target heart rate range for burning fat, caloric requirements). He just wanted to 'get going' so he didn't know how to properly do fat-burning cardio and didn't know how much to eat, in order to burn fat and gain lean mass.

What has happened is that his metabolism has hit a sticking point (a plateau). The idea is that if the body is being pushed beyond its current fitness level (too intense cardio), in attempt to hurry the process up, the metabolism begins to hold onto fat and use the lean mass for energy (kind of a starvation-mode affect).

Solution: Bob needs to get on track by measuring all those numbers (RHR, THR,target heart rate, calories & body composition). Eat 300-500 extra calories every day, for seven days and then recheck body composition on day seven. If the pattern hasn't changed, eat 300-500 calories for another seven days and then recheck body composition. If Bob is further along than three-months of consistent resistance-training, do a 6-8-10 rep range with heavier weights to stimulate the muscles during resistance-training sessions. If you've been training less than three-months consistently, stick with whatever rep range you have been doing and let the extra calories pick up the slack, but base your workouts on your body composition numbers!

Example #4: Gain Lean Mass & Burn Fat:

This is where Bob wants to be!

This is one of the most misunderstood points in fat-loss because people who have skipped one of the (three) parts of nutrition will erroneously conclude that any weight loss is a good thing.

(If they have lost some fat weight while skipping nutrition, they now think they are smarter than their trainer and will attempt to continue working out while skipping one or two parts of the nutrition. By the fifth, sixth or seventh month they'll start getting colds and bugs, experiencing injuries and not make the connection that their trainer told them that skipping nutrition-density, but continuing with ice cream, alcohol, junk food and so on is a stress to the training body.)

Think about it this way: There's only 24-hours in a day. Eight of those will be sleeping time. That leaves 16 hours to get the nutrition put in that your training body needs. If you're spending time eating S.A.D.C.R.A.P. (or willfully withholding the BNBBs), that is taking time away from getting nutrition-density...you'll be going backwards and it will show up in you immune system and performance. Most likely a back, neck or knee injury.

What's more important is what 'trend' has been indicated by how Bob got to this point. If all (three) parts of the nutrition were done correctly, he will be on the fast-track to his first goal of 20% body fat and have a well-established trend, to continue if he wants to be more like 15%, 12%, 10% or less (momentum) by continuing to do what works.

The downside of any habits whether they are building health in or hurting health is that they take on momentum! Regardless of what you think or believe about whole-foods, functional-foods or supplements, your body still requires them!

Isn't that a funny thing? You can say you don't believe in nutrition, but your body still requires it!

One can withhold the very nutrition-density their body requires and convince themselves they don't want to take the time, invest the money or just put the nutrition in even though the body requires them? This is maybe the most common sticking point trainers have with clients (clients insisting they want better results but refusing to eat enough whole-foods, functional-foods and certain supplement at certain times) and being unwilling to experiment long enough with nutrition (simply put it in the body and let nature take over) to see what an amazing difference nutrition makes (80% of the results you get or wish you got has to do with putting nutrition-density in your body).

You see, if Bob skipped steps then he will lose 'weight' for a while, but then the body will put the brakes on the process will amazingly and seemingly miraculously reverse itself, *"I don't know what happened...I started getting fatter!"*

A word on participation in amateur athletics:

As a side note, what commonly happens with people new to fitness or who are getting back on the horse, is that they start looking good, feeling good in months three through six. If this is true, they start thinking about participating in some kind of athletic events. Problem being that if they didn't get their nutrition dialed-in from the get go, by months five through seven their body has been heading in a trend of depletion, meaning they have been using up nutrition more than they have been building it up, especially so if they consciously chose to skip supplementation. Often, by this time they have given themselves permission to drink a little more coffee, alcohol, ice cream, etc...after all, they deserve it! So, they decide to start training with a little more intensity, frequency, duration, etc., but they haven't prepared the body nutritionally. In other words, their ego got involved but instead of using their ego to engage good choices, they used their ego to exercise resistance. Within a month they start gaining body fat, losing lean mass, motivation wanes a little, maybe a cold sneaks in, their muscles aren't recovering and their ego is wondering what happened? In short, they have gone months without adequate nutrition while gradually pushing, asking more of their body, expecting the trend to go one way when they were ignoring the fundamental rule...80% of the benefits you get or miss out on are based on quality, timing, quantity and consistency of nutrition-density...leave no stone unturned.

Just because you don't notice how much body your nutrition is using doesn't mean you can skip it...there's no as gauge that shows your nutritional status as you go (other than the symptoms I tell you about). By the time you realize you're not getting enough nutrition you're already three to six months behind. *-oopsies!*

Back to Bob...

This is key: How Bob lost weight in the beginning determines not how well it goes in the beginning, but rather how well is goes on the back end as he gets closer to his overall goals (you can't fool nature). People often think that the habits/actions that caused initial success means continued success, but in reality, continued success is dependent on the habits that are formed (guidelines herein) in training the metabolism to burn fat for energy (low intensity fat-burning cardio) and simultaneously feeding the lean mass before and after resistance-training workouts.

The person who skips one of the three nutrition parts (whole-foods, functional-foods & certain kinds of supplements at certain times), will be the person down the road complaining why they are gaining fat, even though they are exercising more and wondering why when they are doing things the way they have always done them they are putting on fat at a record rate (not to mention why they are having all sorts of health problems as their body breaks down in *de*-generation: there' simply no way around giving your body adequate nutrition-density and food alone doesn't cut it for active people).

You can predict your future success as well as whether weight loss will be healthy or you'll gain more weight back later, based on how well you apply all three parts of nutrition from the start. Any changes in body composition without the nutrition binds the changes to chance or randomness, since without nutrition the metabolism really isn't functioning correctly. Skipping any of the three-parts of nutrition in the beginning months means you'll be gaining all the fat back, down the road in a few months.

Example #5: Gain Lean Mass AND Gain Fat:

The first of the month rolled around after Bob had been cruising through his program for a few months, when he checked his body composition he found that he had in fact gained lean mass (lean mass was now up to 32% from the original 20%) but he had also unexpectedly gained fat, too!

Remember from Example #1 Bob's body fat started out at 30% and the body fat had decreased as his workouts, efficiency and nutrition got dialed-in, but for whatever reason when he checked his body composition this time, his bodyfat had increased (possibly after losing some fat) and he hadn't reached his ultimate goal of 12% body fat yet.

Since he has a track-record of consistent workouts (both resistance & cardio) and is consistent with the three parts of his nutrition, the adjustment will be pretty easy (since the five-points are in place/three nutrition, resistance and cardio), this eliminates the number of variables and takes the guess work out of what Bob has to do to get his body back onto a trend of burning fat and progressing toward his 12% body fat goal.

Each of the five components emphasizes and amplifies the effects of his efforts; any skipped steps increases the number of possible reasons (variables) why a person might not be getting the results they want...thereby eliminating plateaus or sticking points, making it easy to figure out the next step.

Without checking body comp, RHR, THR, and calorie requirements each month it would be like running your car out of gas and then taking it to a mechanic to diagnose an engine that isn't running well when it isn't running!...without fuel, you can't run the engine to diagnose it. The car can sit there for months and no amount of ego resistance is going to change that if you want your mechanic to diagnose the engine, you have to put fuel in, so your mechanic can hear it running. And truly, I've seen this happen in life...people have trouble with their vehicle and instead of just fueling it up and getting it fixed it sits there for years! Time has stopped out of a resistant ego dynamic. To them, it's more important to be able to make that choice to leave the car un-fueled than to simply fuel it up, get it tuned-up and get on with travels and new adventures. Crazy, I know! When someone wants to be right, more than reach the goals they say they have, that's how it plays out. -Priorities.

So, Bob's body fat had increased a little around month five...

Solution choices:

Do one of the following (again, change one thing and monitor the results for a month).

Option one:

Did Bob start eating more S.A.D.C.R.A.P. as his training progressed?

Often when people have been fairly consistent with their workouts, they give themselves permission to start eating junk food again, thinking their workouts make up for the effects, of nutritionally-deficient foods (fake emotional reward). If this is the case, Bob can get strict again, eliminating S.A.D.C.R.A.P for a month it may be the key to opening up the fat-burning channels again as well as clear out the chemical concoction junk food introduces into the body, which for a number of reasons (there's a few schools of thought and no one can seem to agree why) seems to enable the body to retain fat.

Option two:

Lack of live enzymes?

Raw produce (fruits & veggies) have the opposite affects as S.A.D.C.R.A.P.. Adequate fruits and vegetables contain live enzymes, which make processing cooked food as well as extracting nutrition-density from all sources, thereby enabling the fat-burning process. If Bob has cut back on raw produce, then he can reasonably expect the fat-burning process to slow down. Raw foods do contain nutrition-density but don't deliver a predictable, consistent amount the way certain supplements do...remember, nutrition is a three-part thing.

Option three:

Fat-burning cardio adjusted for current fitness level?

The point of checking your resting heart rate (RHR), when you wake up the first of each month, is that as you get more cardiovascular fitness, so must your target heart rate (60%-70%) be adjusted to reflect your fitness ability for the next month. If you don't check your heart rate and do the Karvonen Method the first of each month, then you effectively miss out on the fat-burning affects, since your body has adjusted/adapted to the previous month's intensity level...that means the cardio is now too low intensity to continue making progress!...doing activity, but missing out on strategic exercise.

Remember? Activity is not exercise! Activity is random and doesn't produce fitness results...an example of this is people who say they have a physically demanding job, so they don't need to exercise, but can't figure out why they keep gaining weight and are hurting all over while lacking energy (nutrition and exercise).

If Bob didn't recheck his RHR and adjust his THR accordingly, based on his current fitness level (this month), he is likely putting in the 20 minutes but isn't conditioning his cardiovascular system nor continuing to improve his metabolic conditioning (fat-burning affect) [doing the same workout month after month without adjusting for current fitness level often causes a backwards affect]. Bob has to get off the lazy-train and get his heart rate numbers figured out and apply it during his next workout...otherwise he is complaining about things he has the power to change, but neglecting personal responsibility and accountability to the goals he insists he so wants.

Example #6: Maintain Lean Mass And Gain Fat:

In the short run (a week or so), this isn't necessarily bad because the body is constantly absorbing, distributing and redistributing nutritional resources to maintain lean mass and burn fat (you have to have put a surplus/reserve of nutritional resources in to get ahead of what your body is using, in order to build lean mass, burn fat and gain optimal fitness). So, that's part of the reason I discourage checking weight or body composition more than once a month (the ups and downs from week to week are not an accurate indicator of progress), until you're getting close (one to two months depending on the type of event or goal) to your goals (in order to fine tune the last bit).

So, in this case, the top two reason why Bob could be maintaining lean mass, but gaining fat is that either he hasn't continued to improve intensity in his resistance-training (most likely amount of weight he is using with good form) or he hasn't continued to check his RHR to establish an accurate fitness adjusted fat-burning cardio (he is working below his fitness level during cardio exercise).

The untrained, naive, impatient person would likely reduce calories thinking their calories are too high, but if they had been adjusting everything the first of each month (target heart rate based on resting heart rate [Karvonen Method] and calories based on body composition) then the calories would be a match for current lean mass and body fat. Reducing calories mid-month would encourage the body to start using lean mass as energy and preserving body fat again.

So, instead of removing calories, increase the intensity of your workouts for three workouts and recheck body composition (don't change calories, until the first of the month, if at all). If these numbers of maintaining lean mass but gaining fat are taken on the first of the month, simply reduce your calories by 300-500 on the days you rest for ten days, as opposed to reducing the calories mid-month when the body is simply going through a temporary, but normal cycle of distributing and redistributing nutritional resources. In other words, don't make semi-permanent changes based on a very short-term, temporary state.

Example #7: Maintain Lean Mass And Maintain Fat:

This pattern is common when someone has adapted to their workouts as much as they are going to within a six to eight-week period (18-24 workouts). This is also common when a person isn't eating enough throughout the day, skipping functional-foods and the B.N.B.B.s.

Bob has been doing a great job with three workouts a week (with a day of rest, in between each workout) and increasing the resistance level on at least some of the exercises, each workout, (in other words, the current exercises are no longer creating stimulus to the nervous and hormone systems to due to the body getting used to them/adaptation).

If he has been doing the same exercises three days per week for eight-weeks, it's time to change the exercises he has been doing. The change can be as simple as going from Nautilus™ Arm Curls with his palms up to using a narrower grip or as different as switching to dumbbell curls...just keep working the same body parts, but work them a little differently.

If he hasn't been consistent with three workouts a week, then there hasn't likely been enough stimulus (to the nervous and hormone systems) to affect change the way he could have, so the changes in fitness have hit a plateau.

The goal being to maximize the 'curve' by getting as many three workouts days per week, during each six to eight-week cycle. Your body will adapt to new exercises based on time, so as long as you're recovering between workouts you want to get as many in during that time period. Doing more than three per week could be too much and doing less than three won't maximize the adaptation process.

If he has been consistent with thee workouts and he has maintained the same lean mass and fat, he will likely estimated too few calories and this is the way his body is telling him nothing will change until he increases his calories (again, by 300-500 calories on the days he works out). Or, he has been skipping functional-foods, which inhibit recovery from exercise.

Example #8: Maintain Lean Mass And Lose Fat (when nearing approaching body fat goal):

On the surface this looks good...Bob lost fat and didn't lose lean mass. But if this trend continues it means his calories are just a little too few to feed lean mass, meaning your cardio is working (target heart rate and intensity dialed-in), but the hardworking muscles, bones, organs, etc., are running a little too low on fuel. He'll likely need an additional 300 calories a day to get ahead of the cycle and allow the lean mass to improve.

Chapter conclusion:

Rule Number One is to make sure you recover from workouts by resting a day in between workouts (M,W,F or Tues, Th, Sat) and drinking adequate functional-foods, based on your goals (e.g. fa-loss, muscle-gain, endurance, etc.).

Rule Number Two is burn fat by doing your fat-burning cardio properly.

If you're losing lean mass, this likely means you're putting in too few calories for the intensity, frequency and/or duration of your workouts. The B.N.B.B.s are a higher priority than calorie-counting and adequate B.N.B.B.s are a higher priority than completely eliminating S.A.D.C.R.A.P.

If you aren't burning fat, your cardio is likely being done incorrectly, or you aren't eating enough whole-foods, functional-foods and B.N.B.B.s.

Most people do it backwards by trying to starve the fat into submission, which enables the body to preserve fat and lose lean mass, which compounds the problems and creates the downward spiral of losing weight/lean mass and then gaining even more back (creating insulin-resistance [diabetes] and enabling the body to store fat but not use it for energy).

Like many things in life, you have to have faith that the system works, commit to eating to fuel the body and make sure your cardio is set for your age and fitness level, so it taps into fat as the primary fuel source, which in turn stabilizes the insulin/blood sugar, which in turn makes the body more sensitive to insulin which in turn makes it so you burn fat even when you're resting and recovering from your workouts...more is NOT better!

All things being equal, if you withhold the B.N.B.B.s then all bets are off...meaning the B.N.B.B.s are responsible for facilitating hundreds of (over-lapping) physiological functions toward your stated goals...if you purposefully or inadvertently withhold supplemental B.N.B.B.s (get your ego out of the way of your success) there's no way to sort out where your physiology is 'off', compensating or under-functioning.(remember the car that's out of gas but they want their mechanic to diagnose the poor running engine?)..*they are that important.*

Like many things in life, nutrition is not rational (we think we're doing the right thing by withholding food to lose weight) or believe we get enough nutrition-density from food alone and that dietary supplements aren't natural, even though the body is giving clear signals the body needs more nutrition-density (blood chemistry off and high body composition): remember; certain kinds of supplements at certain times...'irrational' meaning even though the body needs nutrition we can over-ride the need with our mind, even though its more unhealthy to do so. If you aren't willing to take some supplements to fill in nutritional gaps to simply get a consistent flow of low-level nutrition-density, you won't likely reach and maintain you goals (for many reasons) and won't likely sustain any positive results you do get (big mystery). That's part of what my decades as a fitness professional has shown.

Lack of nutritional-density increases injuries:

One study in 2013 showed that of 52 Division I female athletes, 74% weren't getting enough carbohydrates for their training intensity, duration or frequency and 50% weren't getting enough protein. Lack of nutrition-density increase the risk of injury via lack of recovery from workouts.

http://www.stack.com/2013/12/05/ncaa-nutrition

Important: The body is constantly distributing the nutrition you put in and then re-distributing those resources based on priorities that nature decides on (put the nutrition in and let nature take over). There's no way to track the needs of the body and how nutrition is distributed within all the systems and over-lapping requirements. Nature keeps the body functioning first and foremost, but that means the brain and heart get first-dibs. When a person withholds nutrition-density, the building up of the body can't stay ahead of every need and this shows up as unexpected/unexplainable injuries that can become chronic. The body has to have the B.N.B.B.s to stay ahead of this curve, otherwise by the time an injury or illness show itself, the athlete is already months behind the curve. Sad but true. Its common for people to insist they don't need supplements, as their body is giving them messages that they do, in fact, need to fill in the nutritional gaps.

In 1977 the Anarem Report in conjunction with the Department of Agriculture looked at what 21,500 people ate in a three-day period. Not one person put 100% of the bare minimum amounts of nutritional-density (vitamins A, B1, B2, B6, B12, C, calcium, magnesium, iron or protein), in their body each day, let alone got enough for fitness requirements (magnesium alone is known to be a catalyst, for 300 different enzymatic-actions in the body).

This study was repeated 10 years later (1988) and the results didn't shown much improvements (70% of men and 80% of women weren't getting even two thirds of the minimums, of the B.N.B.B.s).

When the body is lacking in nutritional-density, the blood chemistry will likely be off and the body fat level high/lean mass low. Optimal performance is impossible at this point.

In my book, *50-ish Reasons; Why actively and purposely withholding the B.N.B.B.s from your body is a really bad idea,* (2017), I cover more than 50 things that increase the need for the B.N.B.B.s above the amounts people think they need, including exercise, medication and stress.

What do the bodyfat percentages mean?

Chapter Twelve

What The Body Composition Percentages Represent:

Your first goal, if you aren't already there is to *get your body fat level to 20% or less.*

The closer you are to 30% or the more beyond 30% body fat, the more you have aligned yourself with all the common *de*-generative *dis*-eases we hear about now (heart *dis*-ease, diabetes, cancer, arthritis, pain, obesity and so on). Regardless, whether you look skinny, body composition is one of the main ways to know if your 'size' is healthy or not and what trend you're headed on.

At 20% you're not in the greatest shape yet, but you're getting out of what I refer to as the "Black-forest of chasing symptoms" (where you get a prescription to cover up a symptom which is actually malnutrition), then you need another prescription to cover up the side effects of the first prescription and the process continues, while the person or the medical team insists they don't believe in nutrition or supplements. I've met people who are on up to thirty-prescriptions, insisting they don't understand why they don't feel good. I've also seen the people who begin adding in the B.N.B.B.s ultimately reducing or eliminating most prescriptions (by working closely with their medical team to monitor blood chemistry lab results) and having the doctor say, *"I don't know why it's working, but tell your trainer whatever you're doing, keep doing it!".*

It's important to note that nutrition shouldn't be used to 'treat' *dis*-ease. At the same time, certain supplements at certain times *nourish the cells* the ways nature designed them to and when the body is given what it needs to build healthy cells, *nature takes over* and the body has the best chance to balance out. You shouldn't stop taking medications without working with your medical team, based on what your blood chemistry lab results show, but as your body comes into balance, it's not uncommon for less medication to be needed, especially so for chronic, *de*-generative processes. I've known people who insisted on eliminating prescriptions in exchange for a handful of supplements and I passed on the opportunity to train them (too much ego involved increasing the risk of serious medical emergency).

Yes, I am saying that much of what people go to the doctor for are related to lifestyle; *lack of exercise and nutrition-density*. Some people will always require some medications, but (healthy dietary supplements) have never hurt anyone and often enhance the ability of prescription drugs to do their job.

With this in mind, 20% is a great initial body fat goal. Often, once people get to 20% they feel they look and feel so good they want to go further. It's not uncommon for people to feel like they want to participate in some kind of fitness activity, even if it's doing fund-raiser, fun runs/walks, getting out and hiking, and just having fun.

The lower your body fat the easier it is to do stuff and the better you'll feel (as long as you don't go below 5%). For women, the menstrual cycle and bone density can be interrupted, either from lack of nutrition-density, too low body fat or too high-intensity of exercise, for too long of duration. For a lot of athletes, if the body fat gets too low their energy and strength also wanes, so eliminating all body fat isn't good either. As an athlete, finding your own optimal body fat level is part of the fun (strength-to-weight-ratio). There's a certain point where your strength, endurance and recovery will be maximized and you'll feel dialed-in.

The more endurance oriented the sport activities you choose, the lower you want your body fat (it doesn't make sense to carry body fat [stored energy] that you can't use during the event.

The more contact-sport related activities, the higher you want your body fat to be: football, rugby, etc.

In between is your ideal body fat percentage, often referred to as your personal strength-to-weight-ratio (meaning that sweet spot where your strength, recovery and condition are at their best, but you don't carry excess energy (fat) you can't use during your chosen activities).

Have you noticed some people are very active, hiking, running, walking, etc., but are still relatively fat, unfit and have 'trouble spots' of stubborn body fat? (saddle-bags, pot-belly, body fat greater than 20%, etc.) The most common reasons go back to the fundamentals herein: nutrition-density, improper training heart rate and withholding of calories in attempt to starve the fat into submission.

Priorities:

Believe it or not, *nutrition-density* (B.N.B.B.s) are more important than reduction of calories and elimination of S.A.D.C.R.A.P., for reducing body composition. By increasing your intake of B.N.B.B.s, your calorie consumption will balance out, as with nutrition-density comes a craving for nutritional-dense food! The person who lacks in B.N.B.B.s will have much higher incidence of cravings & calorie-dense foods, in an unconscious attempt to get the nutrition-density the cells are seeking (quantity of nutrition-density should accompany quantity of food, although it doesn't usually make up for lack of nutrition-density).

You can't outrun poor nutrition with any amount of exercise and restricting calories makes the calorie problem worse and compounds the lack of nutrition-density worse.

When you hear people say they don't want to take a handful of pills to get nutrition, this is an example of commercial propaganda. You have to put nutrition-density in your body to maintain your body.

If you don't *put nutrition-density in*, either with food, supplements or hopefully a combination then your body will eventually break down and you'll end up taking handfuls of prescription drugs to cover up the symptoms of not taking a handful of nutritional supplements...the subpar nutrition symptoms will still be going on under the surface, you just won't fully comprehend it.

Remember that any guess (whether by a professional or an app) about how many calories you need is only relevant, for thirty-days (because your body is in a constant state of flux) and is only as good as the results you get in your body composition (numbers you get the first of each month). Calorie predictions are based on averages, not you. The idea of coming up with an initial calorie goal is a starting point that restarts the first of each month.

With that in mind, the one I have used since around 2006 is at this link and is current as of September 2016.

www.dietitian.com/calcbody.php#.UhrpfWS9Kc0

Let's take a look at one person's success story.

Chapter Thirteen

Rob Rector's Success

Rob and I met when we were still teenagers. Back in the day I think I weighed in at about 140 pounds and Rob was about 20 pounds less than that. Rob is really passionate about audio equipment and cycling...those are his *things*. Rob had expressed that he wanted to get back down to about 170-180 pounds, for his upcoming anniversary trip and lean and strong for long bike rides.

He had been as low as 160 pounds at 12% bodyfat in 2011, but to him that seemed a little too clean, to maintain his strength and endurance (strength-to-weight-ratio). Having had prior experience with cycling and burning fat off, Rob had a lot of the big-picture concepts and mindset for discipline, consistency and hard work in place. He did have some questions and we would talk every two to three days, as he progressed with his program and he needed more specific information, to keep progressing and dialing-in his progress.

On February 1st, 2016, Rob was topping out at about 229.6 pounds and 30% body fat (body composition)...about 110 more than when we first met. Rob decided his cardio work would consist of road cycling around his California neighborhoods. To me, Rob is leader...a true role model. He's passionate about living a lean lifestyle and is very generous with his time and understanding of the 'how' and 'what' healthy, sustainable fat-loss means. He is more than willing to do the work and share his discoveries with anyone who asks. Although he gets lots of comments from people about how 'easy' it is for him to get lean, you have to remember that he had gotten up to 230, out-of-shape pounds!

Rob said, *"I want this to work out and I'm motivated to get back to where I was and this time stronger and permanent...as for fitness, I guess I must have been doing some stuff right because a few points you made in the first video (my Be Your Own Personal Trainer video), I have said to people over and over again...I have a lot to learn about nutrition...now you got me thinking about preparing my meals for work...it's easier to eat healthy, if you buy it at the grocery and cook it...".*

Rob started making fruit and protein smoothies to drink throughout the day about this time, he said, *"I am really enjoying eating better and all this. Thank you so much for your help and input."* Rob had some questions about various types of protein powders. I said, *"Well, it's just like audio equipment...you get what you pay for...you can go for quality or quantity, your choice"*. Rob said, *"Makes sense to me. I don't really know what is high-quality when it comes to this stuff. That's why I figured I would ask the expert!...I will check it out ...yeah I think this time around if I focus on my nutrition I will perform better and feel a lot better too...I already feel better just eating better and getting out there on the bike...it is amazing how nutrition can play such a big part of all that...my health is the most important thing, without that, nothing else is really possible...can't enjoy life if you are dead, or close to it...awesome man ...I appreciate all your help."*

As Rob's progress became obvious, people started approaching him and wanting him to use products they were selling. Even other trainers wanted him to train with them. He told them, *"...nah, I will buy the stuff Sov recommends."* I said, *"Yay, honestly Rob, I wouldn't steer you wrong. You won't be disappointed. I promise."* Rob said, *"I know man, and I trust you more than I do anyone out there selling product to just make money."*

I said, *"As a seasoned trainer, I know very well the kinds of comments people make who feel pressured to burn that fat off once and for all. Especially in a work environment, it's easy to slip into status-quo where everyone sits all day, eats for convenience and neglects the exercise part. It's easy when everyone is doing it!"* Rob replied, *"Well, it's like you said. You have been doing this for 25 years and you learn, make mistakes, learn more and modify as you go. Out with the old data, and in with what works."*

By February 15th, Rob was down 4.2 pounds to 225.4 pounds.

Rob is the kind of guy that hears people's excuses and go's about trying to help them wrap their mind around how they can get over their own procrastination patterns and get their nutrition and exercise dialed-in...their "circle-talking"...how to help others have the kind of success he has earned. Even though he is busy riding his bike to work and home, fueling for his longer weekend rides, raising a family and figuring out how to hydrate properly he is still thinking about how to help others who need to lose fat for their own good. Being a team member at major health care company, everyone there knows the stats on obesity, diabetes, heart *disease* and so forth, but as we know, 'knowing' isn't enough nor the same as 'doing'.

I have to say, even after decades of doing this stuff personally and professionally, Rob's follow through with his intent to succeed and doing so within the timeline he selected was inspiring to me. He gave his goals conscientious thought, he believed in his ability to succeed, he monitored his results, as he went along, and he asked questions for clarification as they came up, preventing days of incorrect or inefficient activity. Rob had a lot of the big concepts in place. Mainly, I gave input which comes down to refinement and greater efficiency of things he was doing correctly but could get better results from with some simple fine-tuning.

By February 22nd, Rob was down another 6.2 to 219.2 pounds.

Rob is so considerate in his effort to help others get the kind of success he has earned that he came up with a 5-Step Plan, for helping people get going which I'll share within this chapter, (of course all of this is with Rob's permission). Rob's guidelines are prioritized a little differently than mine, but the difference being that when someone hires me, they want guaranteed results and as a professional trainer you have to preemptively address the way people sabotage themselves, in the beginning months of a program. Rob approaches his suggestions from a real nuts-and-bolts kind of angle whereas I approach it from "do this-get this".

By the last day of February, Rob was down another 4 pounds to 215.2 pounds.

Essentially, Rob started by telling me what he knew to work for sure and which parts his instincts told him he needed more info about...meaning things that kinda' worked before but were maybe challenging to sustain. As you progress through your own program, you'll come up with questions which you might not have even thought of or known of when you first began (e.g. During a 15-minute bike ride, drinking a functional-food drink mix isn't required, water alone is enough. But once you're riding for more than an hour, how do you get enough fuel to keep going without diminishing performance? How do you carry enough fuel with you for the long training sessions?).

Rob was really seeing the reality of his exercise and nutrition efforts by this point. On March 7 he was down another 2.2 pounds to 213 pounds...momentum building!

Rob said, *"I'm trying to do it smarter this time and carry food and eat better, fuel better, perform better...because I can change my mentality on eating I know in the long run I will be stronger and live longer and even go faster... I am experimenting with the smoothies. It's a lot of fun."*

So, we talked big picture, whole-foods, quantity of food, timing of meals and snacks and so forth. We talked about the importance of knowing your resting heart rate, target heart rate, caloric requirements and the importance of 'feeding the muscle' versus 'trying to starve the fat'.

March 14th rolled around and Rob had successfully burned another 2.4 pounds (of fat), reaching 210.6 pounds. During one of our text message sessions, I suggested Rob order a specific type of body composition measuring device on Amazon for about $23 with *Prime*. No nonsense, Rob just clicked on the link and ordered it...exactly what a trainer expects from a motivated client...Rob even started telling others about it.

This device would tell Rob his weight, how much actual body fat he loses versus losing healthy, lean mass like popular fad diets promote. It also makes sure he is gaining lean mass as he progresses and tracks his hydration level before and after his rides to make sure he is getting enough fluid, energy and electrolytes during those rides that last longer than an hour. Any deficit in hydration would cue him as to how much he needs to drink, in the hours after the ride, to make up for what his body used and to assure full recovery in preparation for the next upcoming training session. Rob knew that he would take these numbers and utilize them to help calculate his caloric requirements the first of each month (Without those numbers, any numbers related to calories would be vague guesses. With those numbers, Rob would assure he was burning fat, maintaining or gaining lean mass and moving on with healthy fat-loss that is sustainable).

By March 20th, Rob found he had burned another 3.2 pounds of fat. Rob noticed that his rides went better when he ate more food leading up to his rides (preparation) as well as while recovering and prepping, after his rides for his next upcoming rides and when he ate in ways to 'fuel' during his workouts. We talked about the utmost importance of recovering for a day between exercise sessions to get the most from them (you can't make up for procrastination by trying to do too much in too short of time).

Rob said, *"It's insane ....eat right, train right = results!!"*

I said, *"Hahaha! Ssssshh, it's a secret!'*

"I feel better than I have for a couple years. This is a great feeling," replied Rob. *"If they only knew getting over that hump and the results come and keep coming as long as you keep going."*

Around this time, we touched on the importance of balancing his cardio/cycling with weight training/resistance-training. I did what I could to encourage Rob to get into the gym and do a full-body resistance-training program, which would help him retain lean mass, help injury-proof his body and give him more power/strength during his rides.

It's not uncommon at all for people to feel unfamiliar when beginning a correct, resistance-training program, at the gym...it's a new experience! There's nothing that makes up for the kind of strength and confidence that proper resistance-training provides. Comfort and familiarity comes from three workouts, each week, with a day in between for rest. People who avoid or try to get away, with skipping their resistance-training program cannot even fathom how much benefit they are voluntarily and unwittingly giving up. The cyclist who considers themselves passionate and focused, must include resistance-training if they are to come close to their own potential, with their weekly averages.

Rob explained how he had joined a couple of the corporate chain gyms at different times, but the trainers didn't seem to listen or take his goals and interests into consideration. I explained that's really common and that I hear that a lot.

By March 26 Rob was down another 3.2 pounds of fat. Our conversation picked up about the three-parts of a complete nutrition program and the importance of high quality supplementation: 1) Whole-foods 2) Functional-foods and 3) Certain kinds of specific supplements, at certain times (B.N.B.B.s). I explained how people who think they are so serious, about cycling aren't coming close to their best performance level if they aren't heeding my suggestions on nutrition. Giving nutrition mouth-time (talking but not doing), makes a person who considers themselves serious, look rather silly…pushing the body, but not using the highest quality nutrition? Food is 1/3 of the equation. Whole-foods and eating clean delivers a mere 1/3 the performance, you could be getting. Why would you hold out on your body?

Most people, once they get some level of positive experience from their fitness program start thinking about participating in fun runs, 5ks, 10ks and in Rob's case, 100-mile cycling events (centurions). In these cases, food alone won't provide what the body needs to prevent breakdown, over training, injury, illness etc., so I shared info on how to make good choices about quality supplements, which I've been specializing in for 25 years.

There's always the clients who 'pick-and-choose' which parts of a program make sense them or match their priorities and skip parts that don't make sense to their ego, even though they paid for training. Rob asked me about whether a muti-vitamin was a good idea for him, how to choose one and which ones I use. He also wanted to know which protein powder I use as he *"...didn't know which protein powder to use"*. April 2nd passed and he was down another four pounds to 200.2 pounds.

In April Rob was having to buy new pants belts as there wasn't enough room to keep tightening them anymore. He said, *"It's crazy how much the mental side plays. You have to retrain your mind, too. It is all about self-control when eating and making the right choices...it's odd though, honestly right now, I don't eat as much as I used to, and I don't think about eating. I think we eat for comfort and habit...I can see how people get motivated about fitness and can spend their whole day trying to help others and be motivated about doing things...it truly is a lifestyle...it is amazing, and sad when people don't want to do the work."*

Rob continued making progress as anyone who applies themselves would. On April 7th Rob's numbers showed he had burned another 2.2 pounds, down below 200 to 198 pounds!

Rolling into the summer heat, Rob also wanted to get a good hydration drink to drink while riding, especially for those centurion events. He said, *"I need to work on hydration (during rides) ...I've been trying to find the best thing to drink, the problem is the heat...water is ok, but I think I need more than that...If I can get myself to fuel consistently and obviously with the right fuel I should be able to be stronger and faster."* Rob mentioned a couple things that are 'popular' based on advertising, especially among endurance athletes and I showed him what was missing from the formulas and how that would inhibit his performance during rides.

We talked about the differences between marketing-hype, advertising and legitimate products, with a track record of success that is actually designed to improve overall health. I told Rob about a guy that messages me about once a year wanting to buy a good nutrition product that *"...nobody is making any money off of,"* and I always tell him the same thing: *"..here's what I use and I don't know of any products that no one profits from, otherwise why would they sell them?...seriously!"* (one of the most common excuses potential clients rely on to procrastinate and avoid commitment...worrying too much about what their trainer will gain by helping them, versus focusing on doing what will definitely get them the results they insist they want). Rob and I talked about our experiences with people who want the results we get, say they'll follow through but neither keep their word nor follow through, then complain they didn't get results!

I asked Rob what the difference that made the difference for him? What was the motivator that got him to change the course that gotten him to 230 pounds. By April 15 Rob was down another 3.6 pounds of fat reaching 194.4 pounds at 26% bodyfat! The whole time through the process Rob was monitoring his lean mass to make sure the 'weight' he was losing was actually fat and not lean tissue or bone mass. Without monitoring his food intake, maintaining or gaining lean mass wouldn't be likely as intensely as Rob was training. We talked about bone density, it's significance to long-term health and how to measure as well as improve bone density as you go along.

Rob said, *"I know if I do the right things the right results will come. It might take time, and there might be times when the results are not exactly where I want them, but that probably means I am not 100% doing the right thing. And most people never do 100%, but giving it a consistent effort is all one can ask."*

We picked up where we left off in our conversation about kinds of supplements. Rob said, *"...completely understand and it has to be the right supplements and the right quality...there is a difference and most people aren't willing to do the research to find that out...they just listen to sales person at GNC or wherever...I believe in research and asking questions...choosing the wrong supplement can be life-threatening, like that sh*t from Hawaii."*

(When I was living in Hawaii, numerous people were poisoned by weight loss supplements called OxyElite Pro they bought at GNC marketed as "safe and effective". Ultimately, many people suffered liver damage, some died. The product was banned by the FDA and collected, after 86 people got sick. Today the product is still being marketed online as 'the same great formula").

http://www.huffingtonpost.com/2013/10/03/liver-damage-dietary-supplements_n_4038436.html

http://www.hawaiinewsnow.com/story/23544063/weight-loss-supplement-linked-to-liver-failure

In January 2014, Huffington Post asked why people were ignoring the deadly risks of the diet pill:

http://www.huffingtonpost.com/news/liver-failure-hawaii/

As a side note, it's not uncommon for potential clients who are working through interpersonal relationship problems to insist you help them, but then as a way of working out their own control issues, once you give them the specifics of what to do and how to do it they go and do the exact opposite (presumably as a way of creating a sense of control, even if they don't get the results they say they want, sabotaging their own efforts)...the *pattern being breaking promises and commitments with themselves* that seasoned trainers recognize from a mile away.

This often shows up with the 'gear junkies': they'll take their trainer's ear, repeatedly be coached on how the three-parts of nutrition make up 80% of the results they will get or miss out on then go spend the money on new toys, ignore the nutrition stuff and then complain they aren't getting results, are getting injured and keep getting 'that bug that's going around' so they have to skip their workout...when they do get back to their workouts, they're showing their trainer their new toys and complaining they aren't losing fat fast enough.

By April 22nd Rob was down another 2.4 pounds rounding off at 192 pounds and 25.7% bodyfat. We continued our conversation about the ideas that it's not uncommon in any industry that potential clients fantasize about getting the results that they think they will get if they can just 'talk' to the best expert they can find. The problem is that, until a person congruently solidifies their decision to commit to their goals and do the correct actions, they mistake having conversations with experts as the 'doing' of the actions to reach their goals...obviously it's not. Talking is not doing. If you're pushing your body, you have to provide the B.N.B.B.s, so your body can properly recover.

One of my employers once referred to these people as 'time-gremlins' because they'll take up your time talking, talking, talking and then not take action...as if talking is the 'doing' of exercise and nutrition. This phenomena is common in every industry, but especially so in health and fitness because success is a doing thing, not a talking thing...when people realize their progress is based on them taking correct action consistently, most people regress to watching the game of life from the sidelines saying they have "tried everything and nothing works" or that fat-loss comes easier for others.

One of the ways seasoned trainers, or anyone who has done the work to reach their goals gets 'tipped off' that people are talking instead of doing is when the potential client is provided the information they need to successfully get started, but they keep following up with, *"Yay, but what about this?"* No matter how many questions they have answered comes, *"Yay, but what about this?"* This happens a lot in relation to supplements, where clients seem to be distracted by bright, shiny things (BSTs) and instead of doing what definitely works, take up their time with their trainer emailing, messaging, texting, *"Yay, but have you heard of these supplements? What about these?"* Across the board, seasoned trainers are thinking, *"Yay, how 'bout you just do what I showed you?"*

As I've said before, there's a thousand new supplement companies that pop up each year and most are out of business or forced out of business within the year by the FDA for false claims, hyped-up marketing, poisonous ingredients and contaminants and even products that have no nutrition in them whatsoever, leaving people wondering why they didn't get any measurable results. With 85,000 different supplements on the market, you think I would actually use the same ones for 25 years, if they weren't the best?

The *"Yay, but what do you know about this?"* is a common distraction/procrastination strategy (ADD/OCD), by people who are more committed to not following through than "just doing it"...taking random action but avoiding what definitely works. By April 30th Rob was down another 2.1 pounds of body fat, coming in at 189.9 pounds and 25.2% bodyfat, well on his way to 20%.

The contrarian & polarity responders:

Also known as a polarity-responder, in every industry, there are the people who ask for help from those they deem 'the newest, coolest expert' only to do the very opposite of what their expert suggested. Sometimes referred to as "Fickles" these types 'spend' their time energy talking about what they want, but put more energy into not doing the actions than it would take to simply *doing what definitely works*, to improve performance by 20%. They like to talk about how they have this cool, new trainer under their wing but move from one expert to the next...for them, it's more about 'getting' new experts than doing what it will take to get what they insist they want. Along with this goes the people who have great initial success doing what works, then for whatever reason, stop doing the strategy that got them to their initial goal thinking they'll continue to make progress and even excel at the advanced level...it doesn't work. What works for casual exercise or the initial stages of fitness won't support the body's physiological requirements at the competitive level. Each month that passes, the requirements for the B.N.B.B.s increase. Especially, with cycling, improving endurance, speed, power and recovery are all related to functional-foods and the B.N.B.B.s. Anyone can push the body to it's pre-nutrition limit. If you're just cycling to waste time or go through the motions, or get out of the house then by all means, skip the functional-foods and B.N.B.B.s.

The people who get the fastest as well as sustainable results are the ones who simply do what they are shown to do, rather than making predictable excuses and telling themselves that what their trainer told them to do somehow benefits the trainer more than them or is something other than to help the client achieve their hearts-desires, for the least amount of time, energy and resources.

You can tell where the boundaries of a person's strategy for success is by how close they get to fully attaining their goals...if they do three out of five steps and have had some measurable success along the way you know that just as they reach the boundary of what they unconsciously believe is possible for them, they'll skip one or more of the five steps (resistance-training, cardio, whole foods, functional-foods and certain supplements at certain times), which sabotages/interferes with their ultimate success but matches what they unconsciously believe is possible for them or what they believe they deserve.

Without serious and committed introspection (self-analysis, accountability, follow through) they won't reach or sustain the progress they make without illness, over-training and/or injury. Whatever 'weight' they lose will come back within months. Lack of nutrition-density, B.N.B.B.s enables the body to store fat, regardless how much has been lost in the past.

One of the ways this shows up in real time is when the prospective client asks for specifics on the 'what' and 'how' but then behaves, as if they are doing it as a favor to their trainer, or as if the actions they are supposed to do (resistance-training, fat-burning cardio, whole-foods, functional-foods and certain dietary supplements at certain times), is somehow for the trainer's benefit, not theirs.

From April 5th to May 5th, Rob gained a pound and a half of lean mass, while burning off all that excess body fat and his body mass index had gone from 28 to 26. On May 12th, Rob had lost another 3.6 pounds of fat while retaining his lean mass reaching 186.3 pounds and 24.8% body fat (body composition). I explained how a lot of the products on the market don't provide the performance improvement they are advertised to and how if you're going to put the time and energy and money into your goals, why would anyone get the information and then not act on it? Why would you spend the money on products that only do half what they are advertised to do? Why take a chance?

One of the ways people sabotage themselves and their effort is to get a trainer, but then since they haven't reached their goals before, the information they get seems different than what they think, imagined or are familiar with and (in some ways they think they are smarter than their trainer or at least their behavior looks like that, and they miss out on the kind of performance they could have had if they had simply done what their trainer said to do). Rob said, *"There is a difference between marketing nutrition and fitness to sell your product and what really works...I can't wait to try the stuff you talked about...With GNC, I never really liked that place...something about it never set right with me...you can go to five different stores and ask the same questions and get six different answers."*

May 26th, Rob had lost another nine-tenths of a pound and reached 185.4 pounds. Rob really wanted my professional opinion on supplements and said, *"I also think a lot of those brands are placebos...of course there comes a time where supplements come into effect, but you know more about that than I do."* Rob said he had, *"...taken some supplements that were supposed to help burn fat, years ago, but they didn't do anything except make his heart rate beat fast which made him afraid of any magic pills,"* his friends had been trying to sell him. In fact, one of the companies that had been trying to sell products to him settled a lawsuit in the hundreds of millions of dollars during his effort in the fall of 2016, for false claims/advertising.

I explained how most of the products on the market are hype and don't offer any really health benefit, but I've specialized in good quality supplements for 25 years and guarantee the results of my recommendations.

Rob said, *"Thanks, man, I hear you on the supplements part, I plan to buy some supplement stuff soon from you...I think with your help I can come back stronger than before."*

We talked about how clients, especially the 'gear junkies' will spend money on junk food, ice cream, coffees, alcohol and so on without regard but when it comes to dietary supplements they use their spouse as an excuse why they can't...as if their spouse would condone all the S.A.D.C.R.A.P. and gear shopping, but if they do something that will definitely improve their health the spouse would object? How this shows up is the client asks for clarification of what kind of supplements will get them the best results but then nonchalantly skipping them...your trainer knows! (good indicators or unconscious priorities, values, beliefs and likelihood of long-term success). This is how trainers screen and decide who they'll work with, beyond the initial training evaluations and sessions...which people are the best investment of their time and energy are the ones who follow through and get the best results. Why would any professional trainer want clients who aren't following through and who aren't getting optimal results saying you're their trainer or referring more people who won't follow through?! (hint, hint, clients who don't follow through refer more people who won't follow through).

One of the common complaints rookie-trainers have is getting their clients to comply with the program they design for them...on the flip side of the coin, the most common reasons trainers can't get their clients to believe in them comes down to the trainers not practicing what they preach...in other words, the trainer insisting the client follow a nutrition program but not following through themselves...what it comes down to is the client sensing incongruity on the trainer's part which makes the client think, *"Well, if you aren't doing it, why would I?"*

Rob said, *"I'm very careful to make sure I don't under eat or under nourish myself. One thing I have learned is your need to fuel."* So, we discussed that whole-foods are 1/3 of what your body needs, nutritionally, If you skip functional-foods and the B.N.B.B.s, you aren't even coming close to your performance and feeling your best. You simply can't do it on food alone.

In reflection and comparing the results he was getting now, he said, *"There's so much mis-information available to people nowadays, which can be bad because there is a bunch of B.S. out there...half the doctors I talk to know nothing about nutrition and fitness...people generally want the 'easy fix', but in order to feel well, you have to fuel well!"*

By June 3rd Rob had lost another 2.2 pounds of fat reducing his weight to 183.2 at 24.5% body fat (body composition

Rob had used various fitness trackers and on June 13th he got the Garmin VivoActiv HR which as he described, *"...has the ability to set time alarms to remind me to fuel".* Rob said by this point that *"...he felt like he was getting even stronger."*

In dialing in his caloric requirements and daily intake, Rob compared what a couple different devices and apps suggested and said he was getting each day based on his age, fitness level and activity level...there was as much as 1,600 calorie difference depending which device he used (This shows that regardless how you come up with caloric requirements, the only way to know if it's accurate is to recheck requirements and body composition the first of each month/if you don't you won't know if you're on track, off track or why you have hit a plateau and what to do about it). The calorie counter for calculating average requirements each day, for a month at a time, is listed in the previous chapter.

By June 11th Rob had dropped another 3.3 pounds of fat reaching 179.9 pounds. Mid-June Rob said, *"It looks like I am good to go...I also feel like I am getting stronger on the bike with a few more calories in the system. I am at my goal, so now it is just maintain and build on lowering body fat and increasing muscle mass. And of course getting faster on the bike...which probably will lead to more weight loss...funny how that all works, you move and eat healthy, you lose weight and feel better...Who would have thought???...-Of course after Mexico next week."*

By the 21st of June, Rob was down to 179.2 pounds at 23.8% body composition and by June 24 he was down another two pounds attaining 177.9 pounds...overall, a loss of 52 pounds!

Most people have goal, hire a professional and then see how much they can eliminate from the suggestions, but still get some results...they cut themselves short before they even come close to getting the most from their time, energy and money...they end up having to put in more time, energy and money because they try to cut corners, but calling it "trying everything" (the key word being 'trying' as opposed to 'doing'). Even with his no-nonsense approach, Rob has had similar experiences where people ask for help but then strip the best parts out of the program, but still expect to get results, then say that results come easier for others. I'm certain that as Rob fine-tunes the three parts of his nutrition and resistance exercise he'll be blown away by how good he feels and performs on the long rides, I just know it.

Rob started his fat-loss journey in February and wanted to have most of the fat burned off by his 20th Anniversary for a trip to Mexico, but with the mindset of sustaining the fat-loss, refining his fitness and performing better on the bike. So, the pattern of priorities was health first, fat-loss second, clear timeline for achievement, followed by participation in cycling events and improving overall performance, ultimately getting conditioned to do three centurion races in a one year period (notice he had short-term fat-loss goals, but also looked beyond to sustainability and improving his fitness performance).

As August got underway, Rob described how *"...my jeans were now hanging off me now"*. In February he was wearing 38x32 jeans and now bought 32x32 jeans.

As Rob reached his main goal he asked if he really needed to continue tracking his calories: *"Do I really need to be all crazy focused on calorie consumption?...or should I just focus on eating the right food?"* I explained how he knows what worked to reach his goals, why would he quit doing what he knows definitely worked? ...does he need to go crazy doing it? No! of course not...but if he doesn't track his success how will he know what to adjust when he hits the next plateau, which happens with everyone? More important that calories is putting the B.N.B.B.s in your body...even more important than restricting S.A.D.C.R.A.P.

Rob says he hears a lot of people say they want the kind of results he has gotten but usually say something like, *"I can't do it because of housework, school, family, etc....but the ones that are successful look back and go, "Wow, that wasn't that bad!...just like anything in life...riding my bike seems impossible"...but when you are sitting there eating your after-ride-meal you are like, "That wasn't that bad!...and you get that sense of achievement and that just motivates you for more...it looks easy for me, because I have made it a priority in my life..."* (priority over other things).

"I am working on a short write up of what I've been doing...to share with others and hopefully inspire people...you have to set obtainable goals and with each one you hit it's more motivating you to move forward...the science is there, you just need to know where to find it and understand it...I

laugh at the new fad exercise of the month, or the new fad diet, that everyone jumps on for a couple months, then it fades away," says Rob.

Rob says, *"People are always asking me what I do to lose weight. Well, here are 5 easy steps that I follow. I am not an expert, and yes, I get lazy and have gained weight back over the years. These simple steps have worked for me"*:

Step 1: Buy an Activity tracker - This is not a requirement, but it helps. To me and for most people this is more mental than physical. What it does is it makes you aware. It keeps you focused on moving. Whether it be riding a bike, walking, or running. It just keeps you aware that you need to move. It also can be a huge motivator by helping you set mini goals.

Step 2: Know your numbers. For me I figure out how many calories I need to take in a day (BMR) (Basal Metabolic Rate). I then add my exercise calories to that and subtract my food intake (Step 3). To lose 1 lb/week you need to deficit 500 calories a day, which should be easy if you exercise.

(Remember, the more you restrict calories, the more you're restricting nutrition-density in the diet...hence, the B.N.B.B.s area requirement, to fill in the nutritional gaps).

Step 3: Log your food. By doing this is helps you realize what you are eating, and you also will make choices because you have to write it down. You will say to yourself, *"...if I eat that it will throw my whole day off, or If I eat that, then I will go over my calorie intake for the day."* Be aware of the quality of food you eat, as well as quantity.

Step 4: Exercise. Get up and move. I know not everyone can run a 5k run, or ride a bike 20-miles, or even walk a couple of miles at first. You just need to get up and move and build on whatever it is you chose to do daily.

Step 5: Rest - Recovery is just as important as exercise. So many people make the big mistake of not resting and they just tear their body down.

(Remember, that without adequate functional-foods, the body doesn't come near fully recovering. The scientific definition of recovery is adequate protein and carbohydrate, prior to the post-workout insulin levels decreasing, which occurs especially during the first hour, following exercise.)

June 24th: *"Leaving for Mexico tomorrow...goal is crushed!"* Rob says, *"It's not easy for anyone...it takes effort...anything you want in life you have to make it a priority or it will never happen...I couldn't have done it without your help and input. I appreciate it. I feel better than I have in a long time. THANK YOU, Sov!"*

Now, let's get into the details of nutrition.

Chapter Fourteen

The Basics Of Advanced, Applied, Fitness Nutrition:

"Until we boldly separate the two concepts of food & nutrition, from one another, there will always be confusion, debate and resulting subpar nutrition in the body, resulting in subpar performance and health. The confusion is in "one or the other" (food or dietary supplements?). Food doesn't necessarily provide consistent enough nutrition and nutrition-density isn't necessarily provided by what we call/think of as food." Sov Valentine, September 2016.

What I see as the greatest challenge for people who want to improve their life, is the un-standardized definitions of nutrition. The term nutrition is emotionally evocative *("I'm scared you're going to take away my favorite comfort foods".)* and confusing (what one person means by nutrition is different than what another person means) and is also vastly different from one commercial endeavor to another (whatever book or supplement is popular this month is what people hold, in the front of their mind, even if the idea(s) are actually commercialized malnutrition). People tend to obsess on products that are overtly and repetitively advertised, rather than ones that are proven to show up in the blood stream and provide tangible, scientifically measurable results. You see, there's two main functions of the cells in the body: energy production and detoxification. If a supplement doesn't help either of these two processes, its likely to be a scam and outside the scope of this book.

Much of what people are repeating today is outdated, recycled information that has been proven invalid and incorrect decades ago, but keeps getting repeated as new information.

Because we associate nutrition with deprivation, we block nutrition information out (out of sight, out of mind) *("If I don't know it I can't be held responsible or accountable for it.").*

Unfortunately for the masses, the majority of what we associate as nutrition lacks that same thing: nutrition-density (vitamins, minerals, co-factors, enzymes & unnamed things), (meaning, vitamins and such that haven't been commercially named), so they are withheld from, government standards and subsequently most nutrition standards (meaning, since they haven't been named, people don't get them in their daily routine, as they aren't required to be added back, into the food-chain, after processing, the way a couple of nutrients currently are).

This is where and why, of the benefits of whole-foods come in. Although a weakness of whole-food is a predictable, consistent amounts of needed nutritional components to support life (we usually don't test the food we eat, to prove how much nutrition is in it before we eat it) beyond a sedentary lifestyle, whole-foods have enzymes and things that can't be made artificially. But if you think about it, most cultures have some kind of supplements they add to their diet, which food alone doesn't provide, whether from plant, animal, soil or so forth...think about it.

As early as food began being mass-produced in mills, supplements began being marketed...that's because the nutrient-rich part of plants are removed, fed to livestock to make them healthy (duh), then SOME of the synthetically produced nutrition-density is added back and it's called enriched...it should be called withdrawn.

I was reading an article last night (September 28, 2016), about the cost per 'gram' of the B vitamin known as Biotin. Biotin is the primary vitamin associated with healthy hair, skin and nails, but we need *all* eight of the B vitamins daily (known as B-Complex). The point being that the majority of the Biotin is sold to people who raise livestock to feed to the animals. Without supplementation the animals can suffer with hair, skin and hoof problems...get it?. You can actually Google the cost of ingredients like this, down to the price per gram on national and worldwide trading markets. Last night, I found that the vitamin Biotin is (depending on the hour) ranges from $56 to $255 per ounce, while the price of silver is about $19 per ounce...is this making sense? The body requires fifty or more nutrient factors. Wide spectrum vs high quantity but narrow selection seems to provide better results.

So, in essence we have a culture that is accustomed to having less than optimal nutrition, on a long-term basis, compounded with a mass-media propaganda program to imply adding back the nutrition that was removed from the food is unnatural or extreme, only to have the masses being so used to being malnourished, leading to *de*-generative *dis*-ease that they become dependent on the medications, which cover up the symptoms of malnutrition!!!

This long-term (since the 1800's) program to sell us less and less nutrition and call it enriched goes way beyond the scope of this chapter. The point being that one of the side-affects of long-term, substandard nutrition is difficulty in getting fit and staying that way (adequate nutrition has a stabilizing factor on fitness/80% of the results you get or miss out on are related to the quality, quantity, consistency and timing of the nutrition you put in your body or withhold)...the reason being that without adequate nutrition-density, the energy pathways of the body are one direction (store fat and exhaust the energy of the cells, but not be able to burn fat and feeling tired all the time from the cells not being able to replenish energy with ALL the nutrition (B.N.B.B.s)).

As you remember, I started experimenting with nutrition around age 12. The following B.N.B.B. recommendations come from more than three decades of personal experience and twenty-plus years of professional experiences, helping people get started, get on track, as well as measuring progress (body composition and blood chemistry results), both with and without nutrition of those who simply followed my suggestions versus the people who insist they can reach their goals while withholding nutrition.

The B.N.B.B.s:

The body's first priority is to have adequate, high quality, highly absorbable, easily digestible protein. Worldwide, any discussion of nutrition or malnutrition relates to the quantity of protein any society has available to consume. It's the nutrient that makes or breaks a society based on availability within the soil and ultimately in the food chain.

Because the body can only effectively absorb so much protein at any given time, I think it makes sense to make sure the protein you do consume is of the highest quality and has the highest absorbability...it's not what you put in your body that matters, but how much you absorb of what you put in that counts! Excessive protein isn't any better than a lack of protein, so make sure your protein drink is of the highest, safest quality.

"Skeletal muscle protein synthesis is maximized by 25 to 35 grams of high-quality protein during a meal," says Dr Doug Paddon-Jones, a

professor of nutrition and metabolism at the University of Texas. "Protein synthesis" is basically a fancy way of saying "building and repairing muscle." Exercise creates microtears in your muscles. The harder you work, the more tears. Protein helps repair these tears, causing your muscles to grow bigger and stronger. If your muscles receive fewer than 25 grams of protein in a sitting, however, muscle tears brought on by exercise persist due to lack of building materials (B.N.B.B.s). But, if your muscles receive more than 35 grams of protein, they have all the building materials they need and the protein goes to other parts of your body or into the toilet". (The science of recovering from workouts and events is mainly based on getting protein and carbohydrate back into the muscles, the first and second hours post-activity).

There's no reason to overdose on protein, think more along the lines of frequent (every two to three hours), small servings throughout your waking hours to maximize recover and prevent injuries.

Think averages each day: Nutrition advisor Alan Aragon says that, *"What matters most is your total protein intake throughout the day. Reframe how you think about protein,...instead of eating 60 grams of protein during three meals a day, trying eating 25 to 35 grams of protein four or more times a day. Consume one of these meals within one to two hours pre and post-workout so you cover your bases."*

The magic amount of protein your muscles are capable of absorbing during a meal seems to be about 25 to 35 grams.

Its critically important to separate the two ideas of 'magic pills' and nutrient-dense, dietary supplements. True, there's a heck of a lot more junk products out there that don't produce the results they are advertised to, but that's where I come in. I know the junk from the good stuff. The definitive line is whether or not the supplements get nutrition-density [into your blood stream] or just pass right through your body.

If you definitely get nutrition-density delivered, into your blood stream, above what food alone is providing, you can expect a twenty-percent improvement in recovery from workouts, and events above what you get without certain kinds of dietary supplements at certain times.

Just like a trainer who focuses on cycling has to perform resistance-training, so do supplements have their place in a well-designed and executed program. A part of my expertise is designing supplement programs which I guarantee performance improvement...otherwise, what's the point? With my supplement coaching, I offer a one hundred percent satisfaction guarantee. That's how confident I am that your health and performance will improve. After thirty-years experience, I can offer than confidently. So, when people say they eat ice cream, coffees and alcohol but won't do supplements, I've got nothing for that. Priorities.

Quality and quantity of protein:

Not too much, not excessive protein. Too much can be as bad as not enough. The same way people tend to irrationally withhold food in hopes of starving fat into submission, people will also withhold protein having heard they shouldn't have too much...the problem being they don't know how much is too much, so they phobically withhold and avoid protein and wonder why they can't burn fat or suffer from injuries! Yes, something is off!

Taking a single serving of protein each day supplemental to what food you're eating can be beneficial: Your energy will be higher, your mental focus and attention will be better, cravings reduced, recovery from workouts better and so on.

Ultimately, if someone is phobically withholding nutrition or protein in any way there really isn't anything a personal trainer can do for them, until they get over being compelled to withhold nutrition. I can always tell when a client has actually read my articles about choosing good B.N.B.B.s because if they haven't they go for the cheapest synthetic supplements they can find and say something like, *"I want to perform better than ever"* one day, but the next day say something like, *"Oh, I think I'll just buy the cheapest ones I can find and see what happens"*. Then they don't get results and conclude supplements don't work!...again, the ego and inner-conflict about priorities...results or reasons why.

As you progress in your fitness endeavor, as your lean mass improves and fat reduces, your calorie requirements will increase and so the percentage of protein will increase. Post-workout recovery tends to benefit from whey-based protein (to maximize post-workout insulin response), but since eating excessive animal protein is unnecessary, I suggest a safe, easy to digest plant-based protein, for smoothies and in between meal snacks which doesn't produce any of the ammonia or negative byproducts of animal protein. Worldwide, when the experts talk about nutrition, they are talking about nitrogen (protein). Protein is the most needed nutritional component of the body, but quality and digestibility are more important than quantity. High protein diets aren't safe or healthy.

Secondly:

Secondly, the body requires a wide range of vitamins, minerals, enzymes and co-factors, in order to utilize the protein we eat, so it doesn't just pass through with partial-efficiency (better to eat less overall food, but absorb nutrition at a higher ratio, than to eat a lot more food with less absorption; quality versus quantity).

There's many types of supplemental multivitamins and after 35 years of research and application, I can tell you there are some great multis that really make a difference, but some of the most commonly advertised ones aren't worth the bottle they're in. About a third of the work I do is designing supplement programs for people who want their nutrition program dialed-in, once and for all. I work with people in-person, by phone and email once they are established as a client. People are amazed at how much better they feel and perform.

If you think about it, there's what? -50 or more nutrients in a good multi? Zinc by itself is related to 300 different, overlapping enzymatic actions, in the body and magnesium is also known to be involved in 300 or so actions. Do you really want to take a chance on withholding nutrients that have that much influence over your health on a regular basis? The only way to know you're getting a consistent amount is to take them every day. That way you establish a real-time standard for what your body is capable of and how to get the most from your workouts.

Smithsonian.com published an article by Joseph Stromberg in February 2014.

"Five Vitamins and Supplements That Are Actually Worth Taking":

"Science tells us that taking most vitamins is worthless—but here's a few that buck the trend". A 2008 meta-analysis (a review of a number of studies conducted on the same topic) of 17 randomized, controlled trials concluded that it decreased overall mortality in adults. A 2013 meta-analysis of 42 randomized controlled trials came to the same conclusion. In other words, by randomly deciding which participants took the supplement and which didn't and tightly controlling other variables (thereby reducing the effect of confounding factors), the researchers found that adults who took Vitamin D supplements daily, lived longer than those who didn't. Other research has found that in kids, taking Vitamin D supplements can reduce the chance of catching the flu, and that in older adults, it can improve bone health and reduce the incidence of fractures."

Third:

The next priority by nature and the body is good-fats. Omega-3 oils from fish body is my first pick, but there are some great plant sources too.

Simply put, the ability of the cells to create/distribute energy and detoxify themselves, is based on having enough good-fats!

The brain and nervous system is mostly made of...the good-fats & water! The ability of the nervous system to maintain itself (prevent breakdown) is rooted in having enough good-fats on board each day!

What happens if you withhold what the brain is made of for decades?

Inflammation is thought to be based in inadequate good-fats, as is heart *dis*-ease, obesity and pain.

Fourth:

About 80% of the immune-system feeds off the presupposition that the lower gut is home to good bacteria known as 'flora'. Meaning through the blood and lymph systems, the amount of good bacteria, in the gut affects the rest of the body systems including the skin, whether the immune system is balanced or over-active (autoimmune-disorders) or underactive (infections, viruses, etc.).

Every single system of the body is dependent on a healthy immune system and if you aren't pro-actively adding supplemental pro-biotics to your gut, you're likely missing out. Why take the chance?

Fifth:

The B-Complex vitamins are eight or so water-soluble vitamins that are responsible for pulling energy from food, but also for keeping the nervous system healthy, along with the good-fats. In other words, a deficiency will often show up as aches, pain, lethargy, lack of motivation and so on, but like zinc and magnesium, B-Complex has hundreds of overlapping roles & responsibilities within the body. Knowing that, why would you leave it to chance?

Hair, skin and nails? B-Complex and good-fats.

The funny thing about the B's is that the body doesn't store any extra in the body. Your body uses what it needs from each serving and disposes of the rest. So, you have to put them in daily.

Sixth:

Vitamin C-Complex is another one that we need more of than what food generally provides and different people need different amounts. Vitamin C-Complex is an all-around healer, which shouldn't need too much explanation for fitness-minded people. Again, so many overlapping benefits that enable the body to carry out efficient healing. Connective tissue is rich in collagen (cellular glue), but Vitamin C-Complex is required for healing to be carried out, the way nature intended.

Is there any part of health and fitness that isn't related to healthy connective tissue?

Seventh:

Vitamin E-Complex is known for maximizing oxygenation of the cells through the cardiovascular system, and more specifically preventing abnormal amounts of scar tissue following injury. Without adequate Vitamin E-Complex, on a daily basis, micro-tears and trauma add up to cumulative scar tissue and adhesions which are immobile, contributing to cramping, splinting and stubborn to heal muscles, tendon and ligaments. With adequate Vitamin E-Complex, nature is enabled to lay down enough scar tissue and collagen to heal injury but prevents 'globbing' of random scar tissue [fibrosity/adhesions] (the scar tissue remains mobile and flexible, as you work through injuries rather than becoming tight and restricted, turning into chronic, nagging injuries that prevent progress).

These seven supplements make up what I coined as the B.N.B.B.s. (Basic Nutritional Building Blocks). In other words, these are what your physical body is made out of. Withholding them leads to *de*-generative *dis*-ease processes. Whatever short-term successes you have won't be maintainable as your body uses them up faster (through exercise, training and workouts) than any food alone can provide.

There's about eight types of Vitamin E and the cheap dietary supplements rarely have all of them, so you're looking for a complex that contains a variety of all of them.

How to know the difference they are making is to monitor your body composition and check and recheck your blood chemistry lab results regularly and compare the improvements.

The brain interprets lack of B.N.B.B.s as starvation, but there isn't really a body sensation that people clearly identify as malnourished versus cravings for S.A.D.C.R.A.P. Being fatigued from iron-deficient anemia is one. Bruising and bleeding easily from too little Vitamin C is one. White spots on the nails or lack of taste and smell being a deficiency of zinc. But mostly what happens, the most clearly defined symptoms of lack of nutrition-density, in the brain and body is by watching what your hands grab to consume...the higher amounts and frequency of junk foods the higher the deficiency level of nutrition-density.

Another way to tell is by what you crave. The less nutrition-density in your brain, the more junk food you'll crave. The more close you get to your optimal level of nutrition on board, the more fresh produce and whole-foods you'll crave. Cravings for greasy foods can indicate a shortage of good-fats. Cravings for sweets indicates a lack of B-Complex. Digestive problems point toward pro-biotics. If you seem to be healing slowly or getting injured repetitively protein, higher intake of Vitamins E-Complex and Vitamin C-Complex, may be indicated.

It's common for people to think they have the tiger-by-the-tail, by measuring initial athletic success, performance and good health on initial weight loss success. The truth is it's common for the sedentary body to have some level of surplus of nutrition in a couple areas built up, but the longer one trains, competes or maintains activity the higher the nutritional requirements can go. Meaning, what works to meet nutritional requirements in the beginning isn't enough in the advanced stages and shows up as slower recover and nagging in injuries. It's common for people to think, *"I've never had to supplement before"*, or *"I don't believe in supplements"*, but just because your ego doesn't want to believe it doesn't mean your body doesn't need it.

The part people often miss is that the body itself is changing as you progress through your programs. In fact, after the initial three-months, nutritional requirements increase substantially, to support healthy tissues, habits and lifestyle. I don't think there's any greater factor that inhibits long-term success of health and fitness, than proper and sensible dietary supplementation, but I can't force people to do what they need to do to maintain their success...again, it comes down to whether the person is coachable or not and if they're attempting to work out a power struggle in their life they'll likely skip one or two parts of a complete nutrition program, while they simultaneously maintain coffee, alcohol and ice cream, yet complain they can't get money for their nutrition. The person who is moving through a fad in their life will be overly focused on getting new training 'gear' yet resist applying nutrition (power struggle in themselves).

Conditioning level, resistance to injury and illness and fat-loss should get better and easier with time. If it doesn't, its related to the three parts of nutrition. If you aren't getting the results you want, ask yourself, *"Which part am I skipping or ignoring?"*

Reaching your goals requires lifestyle change...a change in priorities. Setting what you want to do and how you want life to be aside in favor of reaching your goals is often required. The people who don't want their goals to interfere with their current lifestyle rarely reach, let alone maintain success. There's the phenomena of people "just wanting to do one thing their way without considering others" and this often shows up as resistance to doing what's actually needed to reach their goal they insist they want. How this shows up is a person thinking how empowered they would feel to reach a certain level of success, get lean, be able to cycle some distance and so forth. So, they consult an expert who specializes in their area of interest. They'll even start telling people about this amazing new expert they found and referring their friends. But when it comes to them following through they don't...since deep down, it's not about getting the thing but more about the fantasy they had in their head about how achievement would empower them in their imagination...it shows up as wanting people to jump on board, but they skip steps themselves and then blame the trainer/coach/doctor...it wasn't about unequivocal success to being with ...it was about doing something their way even if it meant not doing what it would take to reach their goals.

This is common and can be challenging for new trainers and health care providers to grasp, since trainers tend to think that if they have the correct information, they can help people...but the psyche and motivation is more complicated than that...remember, do the resistance-training and fat-burning cardio, along with the three parts of nutrition and seeming miracles will happen, beyond what you thought you could do...but if you skip any of them (you're smarter than your trainer), you'll have a great 'sense' of control and power (to make up for lack of control or freedom in other areas of your life) but, you won't maintain your success since the unconscious motivation isn't rooted in integrity.

If you don't believe this, look at how many people want to be in the Olympics, but don't make it (a measure of work and effort doesn't assure success, but rather correct, uncontaminated motives). Look at how many people lose weight and gain it back. You have just as much right to fail as succeed and excuses are free.

"Effort doesn't respect what you say you want...physiological performance is dictated by the degree of nutritional surplus...future results are limited by today's nutritional status."

A common side effect of malnourishment is lowering of the goal as a person approaches their intended goal. The malnourished person will lack emotional and psychological stamina, motivation and follow through. As they get a little bit of success they tell themselves, *"This is pretty good, I don't need to work this hard any more...I look pretty good"*. They cut themselves short, ease off the discipline and fail to reach their stated goals.

You can tell if someone is working something else out, if the evidence is showing they need extra nutritional support, but their ego gets in the way and they say on one hand they want to achieve the goal, but then argue and won't even take a simple supplement...they're working something else out (most often relationship stuff/power struggle) and displacing it on their coach/trainer.

Similar dynamics happen with health care providers...people rush to the E.R. for problems resulting from lack of nutrition and exercise, only to spend the whole appointment complaining about the problem, only to refuse to take the doctor's suggestion, leave against medical advice and then return later to complain about the problem, but never doing what is suggested. Sometimes referred to as non-compliance, it comes down to someone wanting something fixed or improved, consulting an expert but then seeming to be like a record stuck on one line of a song they don't take suggestions and keep complaining!

Sometimes, the root of relationship problems is failure to surrender to the relationship itself. If two people get together, but refuse to be reasonable with each other, refuse to give up a part of themselves to gain the relationship a power struggle ensues. The long-term result is two people being a sticks in the mud, eating food and beverage to block out the unhappiness of not getting what they think love is (holding back), followed up with stagnation (weight gain) and stubbornness (refusing to exercise and put adequate nutrition in their body), followed by attempting to regain or get fit, without relinquishing what they perceive as power and control within the relationship (trying to regain control by controlling others, yet demonstrating no emotional control of themselves).

So, they start getting personal training unconsciously thinking they'll gain what they lost through resisting the natural course of love, only to start the same stubborn, resistant pattern or fake independence and autonomy with their trainer (as they get closer to reaching their ultimate goals, it pushes their control buttons and they realize at an unconscious level that by succeeding, they gave up some of the control they had worked so hard to gain). These are the kind of people who are constantly looking for the newest, coolest expert (fickle), but as soon as it comes to them making a change within themselves they start blaming the trainer, doctor, nurses, coaches for not "understanding them" when it really comes down to them not following through.

It's not that cravings mean you're simply making an inconsequential choice of junk food over good, whole-foods. It's that it indicates underlying malnourishment, which points to major health problems of *de*-generative *dis*-ease down the road, since the body has to have adequate nutrition-density, even if you don't notice the indicators. Like thirst and its relationship to hydration, by the time you notice it it's too late. Needing a lot of sleep can indicate the overall view of a wide range of nutrients...remember, chasing a symptom with a single nutrient won't help...put the B.N.B.B.s in and let nature take over.

Let's discuss the all-important necessity of functional-foods.

Chapter Fifteen

Functional-Foods

In case you haven't noticed the nutrition strategy I suggest, there's three parts you want to include to get the most from your program, in order to leave no stone unturned.

Remember that you'll only get so much from your training and workouts if you don't provide the nutrition the body needs. Exercise/training is stimulus for your nervous and endocrine systems, to adapt, but without adequate nutrition, it's like sending an important email to someone and never hearing back (the cycle isn't complete/it won't come full circle). The three parts of what I consider a complete nutrition program are first and foremost, whole-foods. Secondly, functional-foods and third, certain kinds of dietary supplements at certain times.

I'm very opinionated on these points, mainly because of the combination of my personal experiences (the differences that make the differences) and so much time in the trenches training people, who insist they want certain results and monitoring the body composition and blood lab results clients have done, by their medical team. Consistently, the people who skip one or more of the three parts end up complaining they aren't getting results they want in the short-run. Those who get some results in the short-run start falling-short, after three to six months. And yet another group, gets decent results, but have typical health problems that are average for people who have gaps in their nutrition habits.

Functional-foods are products that are engineered specifically to assist the body to get better, faster and more efficient results than whole-food alone is capable of providing (mainly due to how long food takes to digest and be assimilated by the cells and unpredictable, inconsistent amounts of nutrition, depending on the quality of raw materials). Even the highest quality food doesn't provide a *consistent* level or nutrition, that's been proven over and over.

A couple examples of functional-foods would be something like a sports drink which replaces simple, medium, and slow carbohydrates as well as minerals and electrolytes faster than the body uses them up in endurance-type training and events. Once an event or training session goes beyond an hour in duration, water alone will not replace fluid, carbohydrate and electrolytes [fast enough to keep up with use, by the physiology]...hence 'hitting-the-wall' or 'bonking' which, if you've ever seen or experienced it you know how serious it can be. If you aren't familiar with it, athletes look as though they are drunk or drugged when they haven't been adding carbohydrate fuel, minerals and electrolytes and water as a carrier as fast as the body is using them all up. Below is a link to a video that shows some examples:

https://www.youtube.com/watch?v=LKfleTzmK14

Properly-engineered, functional sports drinks make it possible for water and energy to be absorbed MUCH faster and effectively than water alone. This makes it, so water doesn't sit in the gut and provides faster cooling action of the core body temperature. Anybody who doesn't want these benefits either isn't serious, about their success, hasn't trained hard enough to recognize the need or are too malnourished and emotional to 'get it'. Water alone is hyrdating to the physiology, by nature, but the science is done that shows how to get the water into the cells where you'll actually benefit, during the event. Just because water is consumed and inside the body doesn't mean it has made it to the cells where it needs to be. This requires a specific formulation.

As far as coachability of clients, if a person is too stubborn to realize the importance, I simply won't work with them...if they won't follow through on scientific proof of what works best to maximize performance, they'll likely have to work through their inner-conflicts, before they can benefit from true coaching...they're wasting their own time. It's very common for people to seek training and coaching simply to find out if any of their own ideas makes sense, but then only apply what they thought of prior to hiring a trainer (working through validation issues, using their sport to prove their self rightiousness, in other areas of their life). The people who are serious about success, turn their program direction, for the most part, over to their coach.

Specific mixtures:

Just because a product is commercially manufactured and marketed doesn't mean it is producing optimal results. If there isn't enough salt in a hydration drink, the water will settle in the gut but not be absorbed quickly enough to do any good, during the event or workout. If there is too much salt, the drink itself will dehydrate the body, pulling fluid from the muscles to mix, before it can be utilized by the physiology. Water being pulled from the muscles is a form of dehydration and interferes in efficient cooling, of the body.

Example two of functional-foods, is meal drinks which provide a higher and more consistent amount of nutrition-density including protein, carbohydrate, fiber, vitamins and minerals better than food alone will. In this case, affectively stabilizing blood sugar and thereby re-sensitizing the body to insulin, which physiologically enables the body to burn fat at an accelerated rate, without fasting or 'dieting' or starvation habits. More important to fat-loss, than eliminating junk food or restricting calories is adequate nutrition-density (B.N.B.B.s) and stabilization of the blood sugar levels. Remember, I talked about how if you have enough nutrition on board the amount of calories becomes irrelevant? This is an example of what I'm talking about. These kinds of meal shakes can be utilized to add calories as well, for people who want to add lean mass and strength, but the primary focus is on adding nutrition-density with excessive calories while stabilizing insulin/and blood sugar.

Part of the mass confusion is that about 95% of the products that market themselves as functional-foods (foods that serve to elicit specific functions, at specific times, for the body) are labeled and marketed as such, but the ingredients suck so bad they don't really do what they are advertised to do, leaving consumer with a bad taste in their wallet! The average consumer can't tell the good ones from the sucky ones. Because I've been doing this stuff for decades, I know the real stuff from the fake stuff.

Another example of a functional-food is a post-workout recovery drink. The real science shows that by consuming a specific ratio of carbohydrate to protein, within the first two hours after each workout, you maximize the power of insulin, thereby maximizing how well your body recovers after each workout. Recovery being priority number one and being cumulative, how well you recover after each workout determines how well your progress will continue in the days, weeks, months and years down the road...recovery is cumulative...one recovery at a time.

The people who think they are too good, too smart or too cheap for functional-foods are not only missing out on the full benefits of their workouts but they are literally setting themselves up for injury and a breaking down of the body as they go along, which is a big bummer since they often think they are doing so well being consistent with their workouts and seeming to improve, but the truth is you can't fool nature...there's three parts to nutrition.

The people who skip functional-foods are essentially kidding themselves, into thinking they can consistently withhold nutrition, during training and events because they haven't had any problems 'yet'.

Nowadays, part of how I screen who I'll work with, is once I help them design a program and get them going I'm watching to see whether they follow through with all three parts of nutrition. The people who think they are too smart for functional-foods or any of the three parts really aren't serious about succeeding or being healthy in the long run. Anyone can succeed in the first three to six months (simply pushing the body), but after that, as the conditioning improves the body requires higher amounts of nutrition to be able to maintain health. No category of person from first-time trainee to seasoned competitive athlete is above the laws of nature.

Whole-foods are what you put in while preparing for training and events.

Functional-foods are for accelerating fat-loss in a healthy way and increasing performance during training and events of an hour or more in duration and immediately post-workout.

Certain kinds of supplements at certain times (B.N.B.B.s) are taken, with meals to make up for unknown gaps in nutrition.

The people who apply all three parts are telling me month after month how good they feel and how they keep surpassing their personal best, while the people who think they're being smarter by skipping some or all of the three points, continue to wonder why the results always seem out of reach, why they keep getting injured, why they can't get over injuries and why their nagging healthy problems are interfering with their training and workouts (can't seem to get past a plateau). The people who start out relatively healthy generally start having little health problems develop, as their nutritional resources get used up during workouts, which are a stress in and of themselves. I'll certainly chat with people in general about fitness and training, but they won't have me as a trainer if they aren't even going to do what I personally do.

The intensity, duration and frequency of training, exercise and workouts requires optimal nutrition. One of the biggest stumbling blocks for people is when they want to argue, dispute, discuss, debate and so on the 'idea' of dietary supplements and functional-foods, rather than just putting them in and letting nature take over...the proof is in the pudding...when people don't provide enough nutrition for their body, they are essentially saying they know better than nature...they're struggling to come to terms with what they need to do and are having an inner-conflict about what they're willing to do to get what they insist they want. In the early days, I worked to convince and persuade people but found it to be a waste of time and energy. Today, I simply help the people who insist they want to be shown what to 'do' and how to do it...it's up to them to do it, apply it and get results...or not. I've been applying this stuff myself for decades, so I know it works and I know how to show you how to get optimal results. If a client won't do the basic fundamentals I show them, I don't pass on the advanced stuff, so they effectively miss out.

Often, people will say they only eat whole-foods and that's a good thing in one way. Whole-foods have to be the foundation and the bulk of where food comes from. Over the decades, real science has shown that you can, under the right practices preserve the quality of whole-food, but engineer the raw materials in a way (I'm not talking genetically modified, but rather formulated) that functional-foods produce higher performance affects than whole-foods can (time being the limiting factor with food)...essentially concentrate the nutrition-density factors. If you like the results you get from whole-foods, you'll love what supplement recommendations will do for how you look and feel.

Outside of activity lasting less than an hour, whole-foods are fine, but during events time is the limiting factor. Running out of gas (hitting-the-wall) or the brain running out of circulating glucose (bonking) both mean that whatever fuel source the person was using wasn't getting into the blood stream, muscles and liver fast enough to make up for the output of carbohydrates, electrolytes and fluid during the event itself.

In regard to fast fat-loss, while preserving and even gaining lean mass and bone density and improving the blood chemistry markers, ideally you want to stabilize the blood sugar, get enough calories, but not too many, get enough nutritional-density, while hopefully feeling full and not having cravings for S.A.D.C.R.A.P.

For most people the learning curve of learning how to shop, prepare, cook, eat and so on is steep. Functional-food drinks conveniently eliminate the entire learning curve, provide all the above benefits (if they are made correctly), with very little effort re-educating the body and mind what optimal nutrition feels like, so you have quick results and improved health & energy all at once. Properly engineered functional-food drinks can be used as supplemental meals or meals-on-the-go as well. The clients who hire a trainer to help them get the results they want but then behave as if they're too smart or too sophisticated, knowledgeable to use whole-foods, functional-foods AND certain kinds of supplements at certain times, are the first ones to complain they aren't getting results or they don't have the energy they used to. I know trainers who charge the clients who won't get their nutrition dialed-in a higher rate because they know the person isn't going to follow through anyway. The clients who don't intend to stick with it or are getting personal training on a whim aren't actually focused on long-term success so they don't invest in their nutrition...it's clear from the get go. The clients who are too smart for their own good, picking and choosing which parts 'make sense' to them ultimately miss out and wonder why some people are so enthusiastic about their trainer...*nutrition doesn't make rational sense to the under-nourished brain.*

When you get personal training, if you don't apply/do what you're shown to do, you really never develop instincts about how to continue to get amazing results. There's the part your trainer does, the part you as the client does and the parts you do together...it's a 'doing' thing.

Most people don't understand that all factors being the same, even fatigued, if minerals and electrolytes are maintained, the muscles keep firing, regardless of duration of previous exertion. (Fatigue and contractions/relaxation are separate factors). What many people consider the limits of their conditioning is actually missing nutritional factors found in a high-quality, hydration functional-food, drink mix.

Your performance, during the last seconds of an event come down to how well you built up your muscle and liver glycogen, with functional-foods prior to that time.

Let's get into the concept of whole-foods…the foundation of success.

Chapter Sixteen

Whole-foods: *Style Of Eating*

For me, part of the fun of whole-foods is learning and experiencing that each food has a different affect on how the body performs and how you feel in the couple days, following consumption. I personally, as a trainer, don't tell people 'which' foods to eat. Food is too personal for me to make choices for other people. As a trainer and as person who has gone through the process of learning about my body, I expect clients to do the same. There's no short cuts to optimal fitness/performance and what one person feels their best eating will interfere with others.

Additionally, the foods you're capable of eating and making use of is largely determined by how well-nourished you are (how much nutrition-density you consistently have on board: vitamins, minerals, enzymes regardless of what food you eat...nutrition and food are two separate things and should be thought of this way). In other words, the more consistent you are at putting the seven B.N.B.B.s in your body, on a daily basis, the wider range of whole-foods you'll be attracted to, crave and be able to make use of. Read that again: **In other words, the more consistent you are at putting the seven B.N.B.B.s in your body, on a daily basis, the wider range of whole-foods you'll be attracted to, crave and be able to make use of.**

The less nutrition-density (B.N.B.B.s) you take, the more picky your eating will be, the more junk food will be craved/consumed and the greater variety/longer list of whole-foods that are not appealing, to you. You'll likely have (having cravings for healthy, whole-foods requires first to have enough B.N.B.B.s on board...not the other way around). One of the Catch-22's is that we're taught to believe that if we eat whole-foods, we'll crave more whole-foods. But what I've noticed over thirty-plus years, is that the longer a person hasn't had enough nutrition-density in their diet, the harder it is to have break-through where the crave healthy, whole-foods versus S.A.D.C.R.A.P. and junk food...hence, to put the B.N.B.B.s in your body consistently and let nature take over.

The undernourished/malnourished person can't seem to get past the *"...plain, bland, boring tastes of whole-foods,"* (as they describe it) because the emotional-brain/limbic-brain, is so focused on keeping the blood sugar up, regardless of nutritional content. The more nutritionally-deficient a person, the more effortless it is to sit down and eat a whole chocolate bar or bag of chips. Craving for the same few foods over and over is, to me, a clear sign of inadequate nutrition-density, within the body and brain...the reason being is the evidence that the more well-nourished a person (the better they are at putting the B.N.B.B.s in their body on a daily basis) the less they 'fixate' on a limited selection of foods. To crave one food item over and over is like the brain being a song stuck at one spot without awareness it's happening. **The more well-nourished a person, the more 'sampling', 'grazing' and 'curiosity' of variety in the diet is exhibited.** Its neither healthy nor normal to have low variety in the diet and indicates lack of nutrition-density that food alone will not make up for, no matter how much will power a person intends to have.

Will-power is a [function] of a well-nourished, pre-frontal cortex (the very front of the brain where higher-level thinking occurs, separate from emotional-based/limbic thinking) whereas, cravings and emotional-attachment to few foods and being a picky eater indicates that the potentially higher functioning brain is dormant/latent, in relation to food choices and behaviors. People tend to think that will-power is thought-based (dependent on the strength of their personality) or they can force themselves to not eat what they crave or avoid foods that are in conflict with their health and fitness goals & identity. In reality, will-power requires the B.N.B.B.s (nutritional-density) to be in place/experienced *first*...(you can't think yourself out of malnutrition, any more than you can out run poor nutrition with any amount of exercise or think yourself out of dehydration).

One of the clearest outward behavioral indicators of subpar nutrition, on the brain, is when people take offense to being told the truth when they ask for help. **The brain that is stuck in emotional-based functioning versus higher level cognitive thinking will ask the questions and then immediately refute the answer, before consideration or self-reflection (self-reflection is a higher-level function of the frontal brain, but requires optimal nutrition to do so).**

For example, when a client wants to know what they need to do nutritionally, but fixate on the idea they are being told they aren't putting enough nutrition in their body (as if there is something wrong with them), that they are lacking adequate nourishment or that they need to take supplements, to make up for nutritional gaps, in their eating habits. The people who can't get past the 'idea' of what they need to do to reach their goals are the very ones who need that change the most (a reason being that in the absence of nutritional-density, the brain defaults to preoccupation with simplified emotional-based energy and behaviors (defensiveness, arguing, disputing, dismissing, etc.: fixation on sugar/blood glucose even when there isn't enough nutrition-density on board).

The malnourished-person, fixates on an idea and behaves offended or put off (emotional-stuckendness) versus a person who asks what to do, simply does it and monitors the results they get (denotes functioning of the pre-frontal brain: recognizes when someone is helping them vs taking offense to the truth; cognitive rationality).

The people who seem to enjoy arguing or 'debating' the need or validity of nutritional supplements are showing you/demonstrating behavior of the under-nourished brain...the well-nourished brain argues FOR/in favor of nutrition-density, as it notices that itself is functioning better, feels better and feels relieved of the tension that undernourishment creates in most everyone. That's another Catch-22: the brain doesn't necessarily signal that its nutritionally deficient (other than what the hands grab and put in the mouth or the language patterns which reflect divisiveness to the ideas of getting more nutrition-density, in the diet). It seems that the more under-nourished a person gets, the less aware of the symptoms of malnutrition while the fixation on sugar and junk food escalate...self-reflection is a function of the properly nourished pre-frontal cortex.

Unfortunately, in this society, people often mistake/interpret/confuse their compulsion to argue about nutrition (which is rooted in malnourishment) for higher cognitive-functioning, in itself...in reality it's the opposite. One indicator of malnourishment at the brain level is when you hear the person arguing against nutrition or taking supplements...*it's that definitive*...the person who argues against supplementation is effectively exhibiting some signs of poor nutrition.

First and foremost, no matter what pet-model of eating you choose to subscribe the main outcome should be to get enough [nutrition-density] in your daily routine. No matter which diet, book or program you just read or heard about, the limiting factor (the self-imposed sabotage, so to speak) is how much nutrition-density your body is absorbing...did you get that? Just because you're eating whole-foods doesn't mean you're absorbing adequate nutritional-density (those seven nutritional factors I coined the B.N.B.B.s). Without enough of those things in your body and brain on a daily basis, it doesn't matter what the 'name' of the program you're doing is or how new it is....nutritional-density (the B.N.B.B.s) are the limiting factor.

[Eating healthy whole-foods reduces the toxins in the diet, but the consistency of nutritional-density can't be left to chance...you have to consciously put the B.N.B.B.s in your body and let nature take over.]

With that in mind, after getting enough B.N.B.B.s, next comes low-glycemic eating style, meaning choosing and consuming foods which stabilize the blood sugar and re-sensitize the body to insulin. Eating foods that are moderate in protein, carbohydrate and good-fats creates the proper environment, to enable all fitness goals to be accomplished with less time, energy and resources. If I had to suggest a specific program that matches this eating style, I would encourage the Mediterranean diet, as it meets these whole-foods criteria and there are tons of books readily available, on Amazon to make prepping, shopping and food preparation easy.

From a personal trainer's standpoint, a sure way to know someone doesn't intend to follow through on their program is if they insist others tell them which foods to eat. The person who has been willfully choosing to withhold the B.N.B.B.s, shop and consume junk food yet won't even research low glycemic, Mediterranean or buy the B.N.B.B.s is intending to not follow through, by default, blaming the food choices that were forced on them.

Keep eating S.A.D.C.R.A.P.

One other clear indictor of who is likely to follow through is who makes the B.N.B.B.s the first priority, ahead of quitting junk food and counting calories...nutrition-density is more important than initially eliminating junk food or counting calories. Eating junk food is an indicator of malnourishment (lack of the B.N.B.B.s in the brain). One pattern that I have noticed over the decades is that the people who try/intend to quit junk food prior to having enough nutrition-density on board, first will poop-out before their brain chemistry is primed to stop relying on junk food for brain fuel (psychological and emotional dependence). Dependence?

At the opposite end of the spectrum, the people who focus on putting the B.N.B.B.s in their body for at least thirty-days, suffer very little in the way of psychological/emotional withdrawal, since the reason they were drawn to the S.A.D.C.R.A.P. has effectively been preemptively eliminated. Everything to gain and nothing to lose.

If you try to stop junk food before there is enough nutrition-density on board (in the brain) the 'idea' of will-power is rarely effective, noted by how rarely going 'cold-turkey' is effective in the long run...(often people make choices for unhealthy things do to the underlying lack of B.N.B.B.s reflected as cravings)...*the phenomena of thinking thoughts which are inaccurate, yet* not having the resources on board to self-monitor what thought are incorrect...not all thoughts are productive!

Will-power itself is a function of the properly nourished pre-frontal brain...in other words, you can try to trick the brain into thinking there's enough nutritional-density on board (ignore the signs and symptoms of malnutrition), by telling yourself you've gone cold-turkey, but underneath at the chemistry level, the lack of nutrition is still going on...regardless of what you're comfortable believing.

Variety:

Most everyone I know or have seen or read about or even hear about who are really good with the three components of their nutrition plan started out knowing nothing. As long as you're getting the B.N.B.B.s (nutrition-density) in your body each day, you don't have to know everything about every food all at once. Who does?

Most people start out making small changes, generally taking some supplements for an energy boost to hopefully make up for too much junk food and not enough whole-foods. Then they start feeling so much better they get curious and start experimenting with 'better' choices...not perfect choices, just better choices. If you don't go into the fresh produce department and start craving all the colors and variety, you're under-nourished. The idea is that when making shopping choices, simply choose the thing that is a little better than what you would normally choose.

Everyone needs at least five servings of fruits and vegetables each day. Each color or fresh produce has different chemo-protective properties to feed the immune system. Each time you shop for produce, you'll certainly have your favorites, but try a few more different ones and learn a simple recipe to try that particular produce. Little-by-little, you'll expand the variety of nutritional content you're getting and you'll prepare it how you like most. Some models of nutrition show that white produce (cauliflower, garlic, onions, roots, etc.) benefit the white blood cells of the immune system. Black produce (black berries, black beans, etc.) help the kidneys. Yellow foods (peppers, squash, etc.) aid the hormonal system. Red and orange produce are high in antioxidant substances that help with detoxifying and slow premature aging of the cells and so on and so on. So, it's important to get a little bit of wide variety.

What your plate looks like:

Picture a dinner plate. To make this simple, there's four parts to each main meal:

1. Some protein of your choice.

2. Some complex/low-glycemic carbohydrates (yams, whole grains, wild rice, etc.).

3. A handful of raw produce (fruits, vegetables, salad, nuts, seeds, beans).

4. Some cooked vegetables.

This is a very simple way to set your main meals up and how to prepare them in advance as well. Notice, I don't tell you foods you should or shouldn't eat...it's up to you to experiment based on your likes, dislikes and values. Having some raw produce is essential with each meal because the body requires them to get live enzymes so that you can extract energy from the foods you eat. Processed foods have very little to no enzymes.

The cooked vegetables are to encourage preparing and eating a higher volume of vegetables and some vegetables are more nutritious once cooked (Google it).

Complex carbohydrates release energy more slowly and steadily over hours, are much higher in nutrition, higher in fiber (stabilizes blood sugar, re-sensitizes the body to insulin, encourages fat-burning and production of lean mass, helps the body detoxify and so on).

In your first three-months, this 'style' is more important (very, very important) than counting calories. You should take your B.N.B.B.s with at least breakfast and dinner to sensibly make up for gaps in your diet that you aren't aware of. Taking the B.N.B.B.s eliminate cravings, reduce your grocery bill, cost less than whole-foods themselves, are convenient and take no time at all to wash down with water. If you like the results you get from whole-foods, you'll love what you get from my B.N.B.B. suggestions.

Pre-workout meal & hydration:

If your metabolism is on the fast side, you'll eat pretty close right up to workouts. If you tend toward a sluggish metabolism, you'll eat your pre-workout meal with more time between finishing your meal and beginning your workout. Digestion personality has a lot to do with this too, meaning some people tolerate food in the gut, while working out better than others. If you're doing a super, high-intensity anaerobic workout like HIIT workouts or CrossFit™ (which is outside the scope of your first three-months and this book) you would need to let the food clear your gut before beginning your workout otherwise it's all coming back up anyway. The timing of the last meal before your workout is particular to you as long as you have enough fuel on board to get the most from your workout.

Cost consciousness:

It's very common and normal to wonder about how to get the most for your money. In my classes, blog, writings, etc., I talk a lot about getting the most for your time, energy and money. Eating the highest quality foods can be more expensive and requires more preparation than S.A.D.C.R.A.P.. That's one of the motivating factors for eating junk food...it's cheap and convenient!...It's designed that way so you run low on energy and nutrition, crave more and consume it often.

One of the main points I've been instilling throughout the book is that consistency of nutrition-density is more important than eating perfectly all the time...no one eats perfectly all the time. Even I don't eat perfectly all the time...but I do take my B.N.B.B.s everyday, to make up for gaps that are just going to be there anyway.

I've done many comparisons of dietary supplements over the years. When a new client starts with me, helping them get their nutrition program dialed-in, is the *first priority*...that's how I know who is serious and going to follow through. When I was a manager at a GNC store I had a lot of fun comparing labels versus cost, as well as talking with customers when they brought supplements back for a refund, which made them sick or didn't do anything at all.

I can tell you that consumers really can't tell from labels what they are getting or if the cost-to-value-ratio is worth the retail price. I have several articles that go into specifics of this in my blog:

https://sovereign-valentine.mykajabi.com

Even with constant research and experimenting (spending my own money) it took me about a dozen years to get to the bottom of the dietary supplement industry. I can only speak for the supplements I take and have taken for 24 years at the time of this writing, as well as the ones I took from age 12 to 24, but here's a breakdown of how the B.N.B.B.s compare in cost to get the same amount of nutrition from whole-foods alone:

Multi-vitamin/mineral:

If you really think about the cost of fresh produce and consider I'm suggesting making sure you get at least five servings per day, how much would that cost you, simply to get the minimum of some nutrients? The multi-vitamin/mineral I use contains a wide array of nutrition, from no less than twenty-different, whole-food vegetables and fruits for about one-dollar, per day. Think about that. How else can you make sure you get the known and unknown nutrients from whole-foods for $1.00/day, effectively filling in all the nutritional gaps and enabling your body to get the most from your workouts and recovery?

Good-fats:

Like all the other nutrients, the only way you know you're getting enough is to know how much you're putting in each day. Why leave any stone unturned? If you consider that wild salmon can easily run ten bucks a pound and you need a couple servings each week, how much would you be spending to get a small amount of good-fats each day? The one that I use is equal to about 1,500 milligrams of good-fats, for about a buck each day.

B-Complex:

The B vitamins are not stored by the body, nor made by the body for the most part. that means your body needs a consistent, wide array of the B's supplemental to your diet. Your body uses what it needs at the time and then you excrete them through your urine. If we take just one of the B's (Biotin), which has been compared to the price of silver, most manufacturers skimp or leave it out, all-together. Your hair, skin and nails depend on Biotin along with all the other B's for quality and quantity. The number of benefits of all the B's combined is in the hundreds. The one I take has the equivalent biotin in two and a half dozen eggs, but costs forty-cents, versus what 30 eggs cost.

Vitamin C-Complex:

Some nutrients work better when combined with other nutrients and factors. Vitamin C-Complex is this way needing bioflavenoids to maximize absorption. Vitamin C-Complex, like the B's aren't stored, nor manufactured by the body much. The one I use is equal to eating one-and-a-half oranges, every hour for five hours and costs about thirty-cents compared to five organic oranges. Is this making sense?

Vitamin E-Complex:

Vitamin E-Complex is particularly expensive when you consider trying to get enough from food alone. If we consider that one 400 iu capsule of wide spectrum E is equal to eating 55 avocados, not only can you see the cost effectiveness but the reality of trying to eat that many avocados on a daily basis...it's just not practical. Considering a medium avocado has 250 calories, you would have to consume 13,750 calories to get the 400 iu of Vitamin E-Complex...but, with the supplement the cost is thirty-five cents! Does that make sense? Where I live, avocados cost about a buck a piece.

Again, I have to reiterate that I suggest/recommend the basis of your nutrition be from whole-foods. Combined with that supplement your whole-foods, with certain kinds of supplements at certain times. During certain kinds of activity and at specific timing, utilize certain functional-foods to give your body nutrition that food doesn't digest or absorb fast enough to help you during training and events...three parts to applied nutrition for maximum results.

A big part of what I do is help people get their dietary supplement program dialed-in for their goals. My skillset and experience is broad, specific and extensive in these ways. In order to maintain the integrity of this book I'm purposely avoiding talking brands herein, but for my clients I gave specific recommendations, accountability and guarantees of your satisfaction.

Prioritizing:

Without a clear plan (do this), getting your nutritional plan on track from the beginning can be challenging to say the least. A big part of what I do is make it simple for you. Over my thirty-years of personal experience and couple decades of professional experience, I've found that there's a simple structure to follow to get the best results from the get-go. I break the nutrition plan down into 8-week segments, adding and refining from month one on. With this in mind, what I've found to be the most effective, economical and efficient. In my book *Performance Nutrition Training*; (Kindle 2016), I go into greater detail about nutrition, but the big picture looks like this:

If you're adamant about succeeding...

Month One:

Purchase and put the B.N.B.B.s in our body every day (at least the protein and multi-vitamin, but if your budget allows, all seven). Do not attempt to stop eating junk food, coffees, alcohol, sweets, chocolate or anything this first thirty-days. If the supplements you're taking are actually nourishing your cells and getting into your body, the amount of junk food you eat will naturally decrease with time and cravings for whole-foods will increase. Don't attempt 'cold-turkey' or will-power tricks. Remember that will-power is a function of a fully fueled frontal brain, which means by putting the B.N.B.B.s in your body every day, the things that aren't nourishing will naturally wean out of your diet without effort (the more effort it seems to take the more your body needs the B.N.B.B.s). The less nutrition on board, the more cravings for S.A.D.C.R.A.P./junk food will be experienced...there's just no gray area on this (cause and effect). Step One, is to put the B.N.B.B.s in your body from day one. People who try to go cold-turkey without first building up the nutrition-density, in their brain and body tend to 'spin-out' in about three weeks...their cravings kick in, they start binging on junk food and quit working out. That's why I teach to get the B.N.B.B.s in for a month first...I want you to succeed.

At mealtime, eat whatever food you're inclined to eat for meals and snacks, take your B.N.B.B.s, wash them down with plenty of water and then eat whatever S.A.D.C.R.A.P. you want afterward.

(As you keep consistently putting the B.N.B.B.s in your body/as they build up within your brain and body, your tendency toward junk food will naturally diminish on its own).

NOTE: The order that I presented the B.N.B.B.s is the order nature prioritizes use of them by the body. If you take only two, begin with protein and multi-vitamin, but don't skip ahead and only take the good-fats and Vitamin C-Complex, for example. If you can afford four, take the protein, multi, good-fats and pro-biotics and so on...do the order I show you. Whatever you budget for, simply do them consistently so you can accurately assess the benefits you're getting. Low level, wide spectrum nutrition-density is better than taking a high amount of one or two nutrients and that's why protein and multi are priority one and two. Once you have the top four in place (protein, multi, good-fats and pro-biotics THEN you can start adding higher amounts of the nutrients the body uses most. e.g. B-Complex, E-Complex and C-Complex, but not the other way around).

Month Two:

Begin to reduce toxins by simply making 'better' choices for each food item you buy AND begin building the habit of making sure you're getting enough calories, for your goals. In other words, when there's a choice between a candy bar and a meal bar, grab the meal bar. If you have a choice between a banana or a box of cookies, choose the fruit. Successful people simply make choices that are a 'little better' each time (you can calibrate how well-nourished your brain is, by what choices you make; the better nourished the better your choices). If you're craving junk food, sweets, chocolate, caffeine, alcohol, etc., at all, your brain is lacking nutrition-density. In month two, you continue getting and putting the B.N.B.B.s in your body (building a nutritional savings account). Simply put them in and let nature take over. (The psychological and emotional dependence on junk food is a symptom of malnutrition/lack of nutritional-density).

Month Three:

Continue putting the B.N.B.B.s in your body, refining your 'better' choices and making sure you're getting enough calories for your goals. Add in noticing and incrementally adding foods that have more fiber and foods that have good-fats (salmon and avocados for example). If you don't know which food are higher in good-fats, Google 'good-fats'.

Increasing daily fiber:

• The typical serving of fruit is about three grams of fiber.

• The typical serving of vegetable is about four grams of fiber.

• A half cup of beans is about seven grams of fiber.

• A good quality, whole grain bread contains three to five grams of fiber.

• Wasa Bread crackers contain about two grams of fiber each.

Again, don't make huge changes or overdo it. Work to increase your fiber intake by five grams, per week, until you are getting 50 grams of fiber per day (the average in America is about 12 grams per day). IF you start to feel too full in your lower gut, continue with the amount of fiber from the previous week, for one more week and then increase by five-grams, each day the following week. Wild salmon, avocados, tree nuts and seeds, as well as olive and coconut oils are my favorite good-fat foods, but there's more choices available. Pick the ones you like the most.

Month Four:

Continue what you've been doing from the previous three-months, and start learning about how many grams of carbohydrates you need each day to reach and maintain your goals.

Myfitnesspal.com is a great app for seeing what you're eating and how it relates to your goals, with over one million foods listed this app takes the guess work out of eating to get the right ratio or protein, carbohydrates, fats, etc., for your goals. My friend Rob used this as part of his plan to burn off 60 pounds of fat and continue gaining lean mass in a few months.

Month Five:

Continue what you've been doing from the previous four-months, but, begin learning more about how many grams of protein you are getting each day in relation to suggestions to reaching your goals. Protein requirements are higher for active people than for sedentary people. I'm not suggesting mega-dosing on protein, simply getting small, frequent servings (every two to three hours) over the course of the day. Your body composition and performance, as well as energy level, mental clarity and blood sugar stability are directly related to the quality, timing and quantity of protein you consume. Making fruit smoothies (water, yogurt, protein powder and fruit is an easy, tasty way to eat it). Make a blender full and drink it throughout the day. As your lean mass increases and your metabolism improves your requirements for protein increase also.

Months Six and on:

Continue as described. If nothing else, make sure you put the B.N.B.B.s in everyday. By making sure you get the B.N.B.B.s your brain will automatically make better choices for you and eliminate junk foods, without even having to think about it.

Essentially, you want to aim to eat smaller, more frequent meals in order to minimize the spikes in blood sugar which are then accompanied by insulin (spikes and drops in blood sugar is how fat is built and lean mass is lost).

Eating right up until bed time is fine, assuming you're exercising the way I've shown you. The antiquated information about not eating after 7 pm is some of that outdated (almost superstitious) information I've talked about. As long as you aren't eating excessive calories it doesn't matter what time of day you eat (the body requires nutrition during sleep to burn fat and build lean mass). If you don't sleep as well after eating, then don't. I personally eat until bedtime and sometimes even drink a post-workout recovery drink during the night. If people are skipping the B.N.B.B.s then whatever food they are eating won't be getting processed as efficiently and their nutrition-density will be lower anyway, so the point of eating at night would be mute anyway...they're fundamentally off track to begin with.

Preparation:

What successful people know is that preparation is key. That means having your B.N.B.B.s, snacks, and healthy food choices available at all time, regardless where you are (work, school, in the car, on the road, at the gym, etc.). You want to set yourself up so that the choices have been made for you before you are hungry. You can Google "food prep" and see eighty-million photos of how easy it is to make your meals in advance to get the most nutritious foods and have them conveniently at hand to fuel your body in preparation for your next workout. Most of the pictures seen on Google meet the criteria for whole-foods, low-glycemic and nutrient-density, including examples that match the Mediterranean eating system.

The level of your success and consistent improvement is based on how well you prepare...the difference between the people who reach their goals and the ones who don't.

Eat ahead of time:

One of the biggest turning points for me was realizing the difference between eating ahead of time versus trying to make up for the past. Think about what you'll be doing for the next three-hours and eat to fuel for that activity (this stabilizes blood sugar). If you eat after the fact, once the activity is complete and you're starving, you have already gone through a spike in blood sugar and subsequent insulin drop, from the last binge, the blood sugar has bottomed out, the body has begun to use lean mass as energy and you're essentially in reaction mode trying to make up for lost time. So, eat ahead of time. You'll probably notice the difference in how you feel the first day. The brain uses about 25% of the fuel and nutrition-density we consume, but doesn't store much in the way of fuel, within itself. Studying and mental activity uses a lot of calories and nutrition-density in its own right. Eat ahead of activity (preparation).

"You shoulda', coulda' woulda' gotten all you need from food".

Critics of taking certain kinds of dietary supplements at certain times insist that as long as we are "basically healthy and eat a balanced diet" we should get all the nutrition we need from food alone. Like I said, I'm not into trying to convince people. My clients hold me accountable to the results they insist they want and I hold my clients accountable to getting enough nutrition-density, in their body to meet the demands of activity to reach their goals. To me, with about 80% of the population being overweight, not to mention recognizing all the signs and symptoms that no one is eating enough to even get the minimum government standards of nutrition, on a daily basis, I have no idea who these fictional people who are "basically healthy and eating a balanced diet" are. I go by body composition and blood chemistry numbers, not by the way things "should be" if only all food had a consistent level of nutrition!

Two components that contribute to the nutritional confusion is that no one can agree what a balanced diet is, while refusing to categorize the signs and symptoms of subpar nutrition as related to nutrition.

As long as we confuse food with nutrition, the masses will continue to become more under-nourished. Food is not necessarily nutritiously-dense (although it can be) and as long as we consider nagging, chronic, health problems as normal (or even average) we won't as a society make the connection that we're too close to the forest, to see the trees. You simply won't get the most out of your body by providing it the minimum amount of nutrition. If you want to be average, then by all means continue down that path...skip the B.N.B.B.s.

How to get loved ones to take the B.N.B.B.s:

One of the most common questions I get from satisfied clients is how to get their family members to take their B.N.B.B.s. This is kind of a loaded question since you can't make people value their health. You can't make people value something they don't. On top of this, the more malnourished a person's brain, the more they resent the idea of nutrition and in a sense rebel against nutrition. The more a person's behavior demonstrates they need to supplement (cravings, health problems, moodiness, lack of energy, picky eater, sick often, etc.) the more they are attracted to sweets and junk foods and the more they insist they don't 'believe' in supplements...but they believe in continuing excessive chocolate, ice cream, caffeine, sugar, salt, bad-fats and alcohol??

The most reliable and consistent way I know of and have seen work is to NOT talk to the person about taking supplements. NOT try to convince or persuade. Simply take your supplements and drink your smoothies in front of them. When a person is undernourished the part of the brain that knows better (pre-frontal cortex) perceives that arguing and being a stick-in-the-mud is its power position. After all, the undernourished brain is vulnerable...backed into a corner essentially. The undernourished brain is operating out of the emotional area (limbic system) of the brain rather than the reasoning area (pre-frontal cortex). SO, what that means is that the more a person tries to convince a loved one the B.N.B.B.s will help them, the more they resist and the further they get (behaviorally) from taking the B.N.B.B.s to get their nutritional-density levels up.

When the ego is engaged (the undernourished brain is stuck in the ego state out of self-protective mode) arguing, deflecting, dismissing (immediate, emotional gratification) takes precedence over long-term payoff of nutritional health. Not unlike the quick-fix of sugar or chocolate on the mood, it's not uncommon for the undernourished brain to push away the idea of long-term health for the instant fix. (Chocolate might improve the mood, while subpar nutrition continues to go on). BUT, there's a function of the brain that surpasses talking or discussion (I think as a self-protective mechanism) which is watching others do something or seeing something demonstrated that is good for the body...the brain picks up on it and talking about it interferes in the process.

By simply *making sure you take your B.N.B.B.s*, in front of the person, you're giving them the very best chance to get on track. *No matter what*, don't try to convince or discuss the B.N.B.B.s (both functions of the fully fueled pre-frontal cortex) with the undernourished person...demonstrate what will help them without discussing it. It works.

If you want children to take children's B.N.B.B.s, take children's B.N.B.B.s in front of them! The brain notices what is healthier for it, but if you actively try to engage the cognitive (thinking) part of the brain when it isn't fueled enough to respond, it has the opposite/polar effect. Once the brain has some of the B.N.B.B.s on board it's likely the brain will then know the difference and above all else, crave the nutrition-density.

[Eating healthy reduces the toxins which can interfere with optimal health and performance. Eating healthy whole-foods is essential for preventing what we call *de*-generative *dis*-eases. Once the *de*-generative *dis*-ease process has begun (or we are physically active), the time of prevention (eating minimal nutrition-density) has passed/it's not necessarily enough. The B.N.B.B.s consistently provide what food is not capable of consistently providing (makes up for gaps in the diet most everyone has).]

In the Ayurvedic style of health developed thousands-of-years-ago, in India, nutrition-density (the quality, quantity and timing of nutrients) is so significant to health of the physical body that its referred to as Annamaya Kosha: *The body that comes from food* or the sheath of food and/or "made of food-physical matter". In other words, the better your nutrition-density, the better your physical body and the better you'll feel...the nutrition is the limiting factor of the body coming into its full potential or falling short in the process when it counts most.

Recovery, recovery, recovery.

Chapter Seventeen

Fundamentals of Fitness Nutrition
By Maximizing Recovery Between Workouts.

In the big picture, setting up the structure of your eating and supplementation program is a big step (timing). Once you understand how to get the timing right, you fill in the details that are specific to you (foods you prefer, functional-foods that match your goals, etc.). The more nourished you are the more nutritious food you'll be attracted to.

Big Picture:

There's three main parts or segments to consuming nutrition-density:

1. Preparing for your workouts,

2. Functional-fueling during workouts & post-workout and

3. Recovering from your workouts.

These three parts are a continuous cycle. If you workout, at 4 pm on Monday, everything you consume leading up to your workout (regardless how many days it's been since your last workout) is to prepare for your workout to make sure you're properly fueled to get the most from your workout/event. The functional-foods during your workouts (4 pm-5:30-ish pm) are to fuel you properly in that food alone doesn't digest and assimilate fast enough to benefit you during the workout/event itself, without blood sugar crashing/bonking/hitting-the-wall. Immediately and for about two hours after your workouts is critical recovery time in which if you don't make full use of those two hours, you lose the opportunity to do so.

The scientific definition of recovery is maximizing the replacement of protein and carbohydrate in the blood stream, muscles and liver. The first two hours, after activity the body is particularly sensitive to receiving protein and carbohydrate, effectively being pushed into the muscles by the hormone insulin. If you snooze, you lose. After the first hour, the body's ability to respond by absorbing protein and carbohydrates diminishes and drops off, meaning insulin pushes them into the muscles and locks the door. If you delay, the door closes without protein and carbohydrate being delivered and you miss out on the bulk of recovery. Each time you take advantage of this physiological window or ignore it, you're either making the most of your workouts or missing out on it. Your choice...you're either building up the body through proper recovery each workout or allowing the body to breakdown. Colds, flu and virus are a clear sign the body isn't nourished enough to recover fully. There is a specific ratio of carbohydrate-to-protein, that maximizes this 'post-workout insulin response' and whole-foods don't cut it, in the this time-frame for many people. A quality post-workout recovery drink can run about three bucks per serving.

In the above example, every hour from two hours post-workout until the beginning of your next workout is preparatory time to fuel up for your next workout. I've noticed with my clients that the difference between having adequate calories on board leading up to a workout or not equates to about a 50% difference in strength and endurance, on a daily basis. Over time, this represents significant differences in performance. I can help anyone improve their performance by 20%, regardless of their current progress.

Before the body can train frequently enough, train with high enough intensity to reach goals, gain lean mass, gain endurance, burn body fat, have a healthy immune system and have adequate immune functioning these three nutritional components have to be in place. Training and workouts are asking the body to adapt to the stresses places on it versus responding by breaking down. With all other things being equal, a lack of these three nutritional components sets the body up for chronic, nagging injuries that seem to come out of nowhere from an otherwise healthy or even athletically gifted person. Remember food does not equate to nutrition-density. Just like resistance-training and cardio fit the 'idea' of exercise, both are required for different reasons, within the training program.

Whole-foods reduce the amount of toxins in the body, but functional-foods and certain kinds of dietary supplements, at certain times fill in the gaps that we would otherwise be oblivious to, yet wondering why we aren't getting the results we want or recovering from nagging injuries, that don't seem to fit our otherwise healthy vision of ourselves. Without adequate nutrition-density, the body simply can't ration enough nutrition-density between keeping the basic physiological functions going and delegate nutrition-density for injury recovery.

Next level of detail:

So, the cycle is this: prepare, workout, recover.

You simply repeat this cycle.

If you get off track, try to be fueled enough for your next workout and then get back on track with your post-workout recovery drinks; one immediately and another an hour later.

24-hour cycle:

The timing of preparation meals, snacks and recovery drinks on an hourly basis will depend on your schedule and workout times, but should look something like this:

- Awaken in a.m.
- Pre-workout meals
- Workout
- Post-workout recovery drink 1
- Post-workout recovery drink 2
- Post-workout meal
- Snack
- Meal
- Snack
- Meal
- Snack
- Bedtime

The amount of exercise, as described earlier should be enough to stimulate the body (toward) your goal, but holding in mind it's a process that occurs as a results of consistent improvements, not from forcing the body to improve too quickly. It's more important to improve a little bit consistently than to try to force your body to make up for what might be perceived as lost time or attempting to compensate, for past procrastination.

You should feel energized and relaxed after your workouts, like you worked your body but not exhausted per se.

Any measurable weight loss during training or event is fluid loss (dehydration) not fat-loss. Other than extended events, weight loss is fluid loss not fat-loss and needs to be replaced within 24-hours to recover fully. Dehydration interferes in recovery and progress. For each pound lost during a training/workout/event, about sixteen ounces of fluid should be consumed within 24-hours. Hint: If your training or event is more than an hour, you should be consuming the functional-food hydration drink mix even leading up to that critical hour in order to stay ahead of your body's use of fluid, carbohydrate and electrolytes. If you wait, you'll be behind the curve and won't make it up within time before losing performance...water alone is neither safe, nor adequate...hence bonking/hitting-the wall/IV fluid replacements.

The primary concept here is 'cumulative'. Meaning, depending on your values, discipline and follow through habits you're either leaning toward cumulative recovery or cumulative inadequate recovery (over-training). The level of success you get in the short run and long run will be equal to applying these concepts without skipping parts. There's no filler info here just to take up space and if you skip stuff you're the missing out.

Without enough nutrition-density (get used to saying "nutrition-density") as you increase your volume, intensity or duration of exercise the body interprets it as stress and begins to break down (corticoid-atrophy). With enough nutrition-density, the stress hormones are effectively 'buffered' and responds by adapting through decreased body fat, increased lean mass, increased bone density, demonstrable improvements in endurance and strength (recovery).

During activity more than one hour in duration, using your functional-food hydration drink mix, you want to consume 4-6 ounces every 15 minutes. The more your perspiring and/or the more humid the conditions, the more you'll consume, to stay ahead of what your body is using, as you go. At a certain point into the training or event, it's too late to start trying to make up for what your body has used and that generally means if you're feeling thirsty or heating up or feeling low on fuel you're behind...there's no way for water to catch you up at that point during training or an event (bonk/hit-the-wall).

If you tend toward a fast metabolism and feel like you need more protein during the event, consume a serving of the function-food, post-workout recovery drink during the event.

Catch-22's:

One of the paradoxes of nutrition is that it can take three to six months to BEGIN to learn to cook and eat in ways that match your goals. Unfortunately, most people don't last three-months, if they don't have nutrition-density on board from the beginning. This is partly due to having energy to work out, but also that most people come in to a program undernourished and working out only compounds the problem. It's not uncommon at all for people who carry too much fat (stored energy) to be unable to get through their first work out...symptoms of insulin-resistance and energy being stored as fat, but inaccessible for activity.

The more nutrition-density the brain gets from day one, the more attracted we are to nutritious foods we wouldn't otherwise crave, if we didn't have the nutrition on board! When you have enough nutrition-density on board, you'll crave healthy foods versus S.A.D.C.R.A.P. that meets immediate emotionally driven cravings, but interfere with longer-term fitness goals.

People who don't put the B.N.B.B.s in their body, regardless of what they think they 'feel' like eating have little to no desire for healthy, whole-foods...not the other way around (paradox). Without nutrition-density, the blood sugar is unstable, the body is leaning toward insulin-resistance and eating junk food doesn't satisfy the craving, for the junk food itself. The less nutrition in the brain, the more cravings there are for low-nutrition products. Any attraction toward junk food indicates inadequate nutrition-density (sweets, ice cream, candy, alcohol, etc.).

As the level of nutrition-density increases (by consciously overriding rationale not to put the B.N.B.B.s in the body) the desire/cravings for S.A.D.C.R.A.P. and repetitive consumption of the same foods decreases while performance levels increase and motivation and will-power go off the charts. That's part of the reason that nutrition-density makes up 80% of the results you get or miss out on.

Rest:

Between workouts, you have to get enough sleep. Sleep is when many of the physiological adaptations like burning fat and gaining muscle occur (not so much during training itself). The less sleep you get, the higher your stress hormones will be which interfere with fitness/athletic progress. Everyone's sleep requirements are unique to them.

Let's talk about the most common sticking points.

Chapter Eighteen

Common Sticking Points

One of my favorite television shows is *The Dog Whisperer*. Not only do I love dogs, I love that Cesar Milan gets to the heart of matters to help dogs that are often labeled as dangerous to themselves, others and society...often helping dogs that can't seem to be helped (I rescued a pit bull in Seattle and know exactly how much work it can be. Sweetie lived with us for twelve-and-a-half years). Cesar does get some criticism from animal rights organizations but having worked with dogs, horses and cows a lot I can tell you he doesn't hurt the animals, but helps them work through sticking points in their psyche, which have often been created/enabled and reinforced by humans with good intention. If one thinks that working through emotional or psychological sticking points is abusive then I don't know what to say!

Take a dog that has a fear of walking across a shiny floor. You can talk with the dog, pick it up and carry it, push it, pull it and ultimately the dog has to walk across the floor and build in a base of experience that is contrary to it fear or 'belief' (so to speak) that the floor is somehow scary or dangerous. In the initial process of showing the dog it can do it, the dog may freeze up, resist, shake, lay down, growl, urinate, and even act catatonic. Some dog behavioral cases are solved within a couple minutes (in amazement of the dog owners) and some might take close to an hour. Some cases require follow up and some are so serious (where aggression is a factor) the dog has to go to Cesar's Dog Psychology Center for weeks to sort of detoxify and learn healthier social behaviors with other dogs who have also been socialized and rehabilitated. The show has been airing for years so there's a lot of material and examples there. The point being that talking about accomplishing something and actually doing it are too different things. If we go back to the dog afraid of the floor (dysfunction), ultimately the dog has to experience safe experiences on the floor before the old programming will have less of a hold...then the new success has to be repeated. If Cesar tried to help the dog the same way everyone else tried to help the dog he would likely get a similar result with little relief for the phobic dog...we already know what doesn't work!

Cesar tends to take a psychological approach versus an emotional approach (hint, hint) and gets seemingly miraculous results few other dog trainers (if any) achieve. The point being, that in that moment just before the dog realizes it doesn't have to be scared...that it is safe on the floor, it does everything it knows to do to manipulate its environment, to not cross the floor...avoiding that point right before it finds the resistance wasn't the only possible reality. In order to really integrate the experience, the dog might shake, shiver, wine and pull away...not at all unlike humans in psychological therapy before they have break through. It's just that most of the examples of dog owners see the resistance right before resolution and conclude it must be harmful and back off, right before the dog would psychologically heal (lack of follow through/hint, hint).

In one episode, Cesar said in describing that moment right before break through happens like this, *"You have to go through that, to get past that"*.

In other words, the dog wouldn't have resolution and integration if they didn't get to the point where they felt like they couldn't motivate themselves to cross the floor and then do it anyway. Fear, masked by lack of motivation is first and foremost to protect us from hurting ourselves and if we only had a primal brain or brain stem like an alligator that might be enough. But the point of having a pre-frontal cortex of the brain is to be able to rationally (separate from emotions/higher cognitive thinking) to think about our thoughts!

I had similar experiences when I first started learning to fly helicopters. It had been a lifelong goal for me to fly, but the first couple weeks of flight school my legs were shaking so much, when walking out to the flight line, I wasn't sure I could stand up! But I just kept moving forward one step at a time. I pushed through the fear to get the payoff of reaching my goal to fly helicopters. Of course, with time my legs didn't shake anymore. The part that changed was me.

People who are stuck aren't thinking about their thoughts nor backing up rational thought with correct action! They're simply having a feeling without examining them, then avoiding action which takes them right to the point of having breakthrough, essentially unwittingly carrying emotional baggage that no longer serves them.

Truthfully, when people simply follow the guidelines herein they get what they and their circle of influence consider amazing and satisfying results.

But even though it is that simple, every area of endeavor has the people who simply set a goal, figure out what hoops they have to jump through (the work) and then go to work to completion. Every endeavor also has the people who see the people doing the work and getting the results, say they want those same results but then have a seemingly endless and ever expanding list of why they are different, why the rules of nature don't apply to them, why they are the one and only exception to science, why they have to pick the program apart until there's nothing left that resembles strategy for success or the model of success and then complain the program isn't providing the implied results.

Coachable?

Ultimately, you can narrow down progress or lack thereof as two primary categories: coachable and non-coachable individuals, meaning coachable people who want to absorb the information to get where they say they want to go and people who won't take in anything provided to them, accompanied by excuses, defensiveness, overly sensitivity and a victim, wounded mentality.

One of the most common behaviors that shows up like this for professional trainers and coaches is when people insist they want to get 'training' but they don't want to lose weight. That would be like saying you want to run but not efficiently or like you want to get strong but not 'that' strong. When you hear that kind of statement, either from yourself or others, it's pointing to lack of commitment, apprehension, accountability and willingness to be coached. How this comes about is a person lacking in discipline to get where they want to be in their own life, get themselves out of shape and off track, but then instead of taking in the information that will help them get what they insist they want, the take a polarity response (opposite) and develop a defense-based, coping mechanism because they feel they can't handle constructive criticism from the person they paid to help them! When you see a person who definitely needs to burn fat for their own good, but says something like, *"I just want to get in shape but I don't want to focus on losing weight,"* that's what's going on. Yes, health should come first and be a higher priority than losing weight at any cost, but when the client or athlete says it that way, it points to defensiveness and insecurity more than a priority on health.

In cases like this where the person is lacking in personality development they misinterpret coaching/training as criticism and ultimately block out the very information they need to succeed, blocking the information others are using to succeed efficiently. To the trainer or coach, when you have a client or even meet someone on the street like this it feels like you're talking to a brick wall...effort just to have a conversation. When you coach a coachable person, they absorb the information so readily, it feels like it's being sucked off of you. The coachable person will say, *"You won't believe what happened,"* while the non coachable person will say, *"I've tried everything and nothing worked"*. In reality, they have tried everything to not change or let good information change their failure strategy and succeeded at that very well! They're using the energy they could have used to succeed to prevent success!

The follow up to this kind of personality is where they pick and choose which 'part' of the program they will do, then insist the program isn't working. Imagine a competitive athlete telling the coach they aren't going to participate in all the training, but they expect to get full credit when the team succeeds and you can hear the arrogance (fear and anger) combined with entitlement (do it for me; *"I'm not strong enough to be told the correct way, but want credit anyway."*) within their belief systems.

One of my favorites that I can hear coming from a mile away is people who are using excuses as their primary strategy will say, *"I just need to do such and such..."* followed by, *"...then I have to ...but first I have to..."* and along comes a barrage of actions that supposedly need to be done, but each subsequent action is dependent on finishing the prior action, which is procrastinated out of feeling overwhelmed, by all the possibilities.

The excuse is covering up the underlying thing which is cognitively (of thought) interfering with physical action. Successful fitness enthusiasts and athletes recognize the pattern...it sticks out like a sore thumb because anything other than simply doing the actions is excuses based /rooted in the cognitive problem which distracts from physical activity.

The people who say they have struggled with, say weight loss for decades as though it's a mystery, but then they immediately follow that up with, *"I just need to..."* as if this one thing the name is their expert opinion of why it has never worked before. If they knew what the thing was that they had to do, they would have done it. In actuality, what is happening is the thing they need to do is 'encoded' (outside their own conscious awareness) and they call it something else...so the thing they call it, actually isn't the thing at all that needs to be done and that's why doing it never produced the results they say it will (by encoding it/calling it something else, the emotional pain that is the root of the problem state is effectively blocked/suppressed away from the conscious awareness).

Regardless of what someone insists they need to do to reach their goals, simply doing the exercise and nutrition produces the results...everything else is just talk. How to know which category you're in, is if you say what you want, but then won't follow through with what's suggested...*kidding yourself.*

Often, reaching goals is more about setting aside the traits and habits which are inhibiting success, more than trying to build new ones. It's not uncommon that when someone has set a new goal in one area of their life they are actually trying to solve a problem in another area of their life, but for whatever reason they don't feel they can work on that area directly...so what you'll see and hear in yourself and others, is insistence on achieving the goal, consulting the expert of their choice but then refusing to do what it takes backed up by excuses.

The point being that they are trying to indirectly work out the other problem (often struggling with the natural laws of nature) imagining that if they can just "do this thing their way" everything will be ok. The problem being that they don't understand yet that doing things 'their way' doesn't assure success and speaks of trying to reinvent the wheel. For the people who truly just want to reach the goal the simply do what works. If someone thinks their input will somehow change the laws of nature, they'll do everything but what works then complain nothing works!

[Success is often neither being right nor wrong...it's state that emerges as a cooperative effect between coach/trainer, client/athlete, body/laws of nature. The person who has to be 'right' won't surrender to the process within the work and effort and end up being too tense to allow the success to happen, often experiencing maladaptive tension patterns in the body showing up as nagging injuries, which jump from one area to another without apparent cause.]

As a body-worker, I recognized that every person has a pattern and place they store tension in the body. There certainly are common patterns like people storing stress in the neck and upper back, but that's a very base/basic pattern (pain in the neck). The more complex patterns are the ones where anxiety, fear and sadness (versus stress) are stored within a muscle group and interfere with proper function, flexibility, range of motion and power (nagging injury).

Exercise itself can be a barometer of which area of the body is the weakest link. There is the physical strength/weakness that is easy to recognize, but once you've got a solid base and experience at conditioning, injuries that occur as a mature athlete are more related to nutrition deficiency that is outside your awareness (*"I think I eat really good."*), or the emotional components showing up as weakness, instability, tightness, etc. It's not uncommon for the nutritionally-deficient athlete to think they are having an "off day" (it happens) but, if the three parts of nutrition aren't being applied every day, "off days" are more common than they need to be in relation to simply recovering.

Also, in every endeavor are the professionals who have already done all the research to find what works, what doesn't and why. In every professional arena there are the experts who know how to get results, how to measure progress and how to know what to do if a client isn't getting results and how to diagnose why the client isn't getting results. In other words, seasoned professionals can often predict, from the first conversation, which self-sabotage strategies the client will most likely attempt to rely on as the reasons why the program isn't working for them. Often, due to various forms of self-absorption, what clients don't realize is that professionals have already heard every excuse there is...any delusion about the connection between hard, smart, consistent work and results is only in the mind of the client. In other words, do the work, get the results!

Thinking and saying vs doing:

The results of exercise and nutrition come from doing, not talking about doing nor thinking about doing. Maybe the most common sticking point for the population is mistaking talking about working out and getting nutrition for actually doing the work. It's not uncommon at all for people to insist they are doing a program the way it was demonstrated, but when checked by their trainer find they weren't doing any single part of the program correctly. This brings up the value of actually having a trainer for correct form and accountability. **When I started working out my trainer designed my program six to eight-weeks, at a time, but I performed all the exercises on my own.**

Lack of interest:

I think it goes without saying that again, no matter the area of interest, if you want to get good at something you have to be genuinely interested and passionate about the end result, first and foremost, but also the process itself in a day-in, day-out basis. One of the common sticking points in fitness and athletics is lack of attention, focus and/or interest in the topic. Whatever you want to get good at you'll be spending significant time and energy improving your efficiency at the program you're doing toward your goal. A point of caution here: This does NOT mean thinking and imagining ways to change the program fundamentals to fit what your previous lifestyle was or what seems comfortable or familiar. The point is to invest your time figuring out how you'll manage your time, energy and resources to fit the program into your life. If at any point you're trying to figure which parts of the program you can skip, you're wrong...you'll be one of the people who say they're doing everything, but not getting the results...(investing energy avoiding either the three parts of nutrition, the resistance-training or the cardio is not the same as actually doing all five). This is a reason why most of the population is so unhealthy...so much work and attention put toward avoiding doing the work vs simply doing the work.

If you aren't spending time fitting the program into your life you won't get the results (at anything you do).

The emotions:

And that is a great lead in to a little bit about emotions and how they can sabotage success. In my book, *Weighting To Wait; The Emotions of Permanent Weight Loss* (Amazon Kindle, 2016), I cover just about every aspect I've ever seen when it comes to people allowing their emotions to control them and ultimately sabotage their fitness/fat-loss efforts versus using the emotions as a catalyst for success.

In most simple terms, if you're talking, figuring, thinking and imagining (procrastinating), more than simply doing the actions, its highly likely you're allowing your emotions to run you rather than being in a highly productive, inspiring, motivated state the majority of the time. Thinking and talking (making excuses and having reasons why you aren't doing) are symptoms of being emotionally-stuck. Doing (simply doing the actions without making up excuses or picking a program apart) is an example of using your emotions to fuel your progress and move you toward your goal completion one day at a time.

When people ask, *"How do I stay motivated?"*, they are effectively telling the world they're using their emotions inappropriately, for their goals they say they want...they aren't taking responsibility for using their mind, leaving it rather to chance and the payoff of avoiding work in the long run for the immediate satisfaction of not following through in the moment.

Perspective on self and locus of focus (what you focus on increases):

It is certainly common that people don't know what they don't know...*self-awareness, self-knowledge, introspection.*

There are many ways to know how to know if you need to do some personal development work, before you'll make it to the next level of your success.

One of the most common indicators of self-sabotage is when you hear or see yourself complaining about how others have disappointed you, let you down or not done enough for you, but you have effectively been repeating the same patterns in your own life. A red flag, to this phenomena, is when a person is constantly saying they aren't getting enough emotional-support. First and foremost, if you aren't developing and cultivating your own emotional-fortitude, others aren't going to give you more emotional-support. It's kind of like wealthy people being given gifts and so forth. When you seem to be well-off, people want to reward that behavior.

On the other hand, if you seem emotionally-deficient, you come across as needy and people avoid, steer clear and withhold from emotionally needy people. People can tell how emotionally-balanced, effective or responsible you are by the words that come out of your mouth...so you have to listen to what you are saying...what messages you are repeating. The most common indicator of emotional abundance/deficiency is people who constantly repeat they don't have enough support. By repeating this, you'll at first attract people who feel sorry for you or sympathize, but if you don't take what they give and cultivate it into more emotional integrity...cultivate in yourself into what you insist you want, people will get tired and recognize it as simple complaining and venting...pointless energy designed to gain sympathy. Anyone attracted by complaining will likely be a complainer themselves...you can't solve a problem with the same thinking that created the problem!

If on the other hand, you give positive energy to others and lift them up, you'll likely find yourself surrounded by admirers, regardless your level of fitness/athletic development...you get what you give, not you get what you think you need.

Self-reflection:

Self-reflection is a process of looking at yourself from the outside, as though you're watching someone else, and objectively analyzing how you invest/spend your time, energy and resources...having some level of objectivity. If you can't look at your challenges from different angles other than first-person subjectivity, you'll likely remain passive, disempowered and as though the world happens 'to you', potentially cut off from your personal power. The quality of people you associate with is included in this. Studies have shown that your body composition as well as your income level will be the average of the five people you associate with the most...lifestyle and habits determine quality of life, so you have to be careful about the values, motives and agenda of those you consider.

Who you attract is directly associated with what you choose to talk about. If you habitually complain about your problems, some of who you'll attract will also be other disempowered individuals, people who want to take advantage of people with a victim mentality or simply people who want to you to listen to them complain.

Complaining implies weakness.

Some people are born into success-oriented families, where the obvious and not so obvious life skills, coping skills, family skills, financial skills, healthy & fitness skills, social and otherwise are inherent, from the beginning, as if they are built into each generation, without thought.

On the other hand, some people are born into family where it's as though they are behind the eight-ball, from day one, having to deal with dysfunction, addiction, co-dependency, poverty mindset, reactive vs proactive coping habits, lack of health & fitness habits and so on...it' the luck of the draw.

The common denominator among all people who reach their goals in health & fitness (regardless where they started from or the quality of life prior) is that they simply do the workouts, do all three parts of the nutrition, notice where they want to improve themselves next and avoid self-criticism, but rather make changes to improve on a constant and continual basis (no one knows everything when they begin) without making excuses, without trying to talk their way out of the work, but rather using their emotional-motivation to move toward what they want proactively...they get results often having not told anyone about their goals, leaving no room for excuses and no room to be talked out of their intentions...leaving no room for 'talk', but rather 'doing'.

Often in these cases, people seem to make such drastic changes in their healthy appearance, within months, that they shock those around them who can't understand that it simply comes down to an effective exercise program, performed three days per week, backed up by a complete nutrition program.

The people who are the most stuck in inaction will do well, looking back at what true roles models behaved like in their early years. If mom didn't wash dishes, then make sure the dishes are washed! If mom didn't put laundry away, put it away! If mom didn't exercise by all means you know where the idea and belief that supports lack of exercise comes from! Exercise! This isn't to say blame needs to be placed, it's just that it's common sense we learn behaviors from those around us before we even know we are learning! Sometimes the problem state is just outside the awareness because we learned to copy it before we even knew we were being shown something. It's not uncommon for one person in a family to want to break out of the mold and demand a higher quality of life, only to have more programming that inhibits them and have no idea what they need to do to reach their goals. It's also not uncommon to have to work through the conflicts of who they learned to be versus who they now want to become.

Priorities:

You have to make space in your schedule that nothing can interfere with. That is time for resistance-training, cardio and the three parts of nutrition. No one is going to do it for you. You have to literally build this into your schedule and not let anything interfere with it. If you don't then you don't want it bad enough.

Interference:

Across the board, with all things being equal, the factor behind attitude which inhibits progress the most is recreational drugs. There's just something about the clients who give themselves permission to do drugs and insist the drugs aren't interfering in any way. It's common for addicts to insist the fitness components are interfering with their social life or lifestyle in general. Trainers see these folks working out, being very active but not having much in the way improvements in their body/body composition. If you really think about it, there's 168 hours in a week. Figure 56 hours for sleep. Four hours for exercise. That leaves about 108 hours to put nutrition in the body. Eating healthy takes time. There really isn't time to do drugs and get enough nutrition to fuel your body. If you have addiction issues going on, you'll have to address those before reasonably expecting to get much value from your workouts. If you're in denial about it, that's your prerogative.

Unhealthy relationships:

The quality of people you have in your life has a direct-affect, on how easy it is to stay on track with resistance, cardio and nutrition.

Co-dependency is the tendency for a person to prioritize themselves and their self-care/health lower than those they consider important in their life. Meaning, they take care of what others want and feel, first and they get what's left over. Constant attentiveness to others' emotions and well-being is a symptom of co-dependency and its very common for personal training clients to think that they can continue taking care of others more than themselves yet be physically, mentally, emotionally and spiritually healthy. Emotionally needing a 'place' and a 'role' is a common reason for taking care of others over self.

Chronic health problems are often related to taking too much care of others and deprioritizing themselves. A common factor in this scenario is when a person's identity is that of care taker to other family members, even if the others are their parents (role reversal). Constant attentiveness to others' emotions can be emotionally-draining for the care taker, even if they insist they like it. Codependency and addiction go hand in hand, much addiction being rooted in co-dependent relationships. You may hear a person say they have been doing everything for other and now they are doing 'this' for themselves, but as long as they are maintaining the codependency it's very difficult (unlikely) to create clear enough boundaries to really take care of themselves. Truly helping others by setting the example that as adults, we can take care of ourselves rather than making other dependant on us is more empowering to others, than doing everything for them. Counseling/therapy/12-Step programs are indicated to establish healthy relationships and healthy priority of self.

Unsupportive friends, family and influencers can potentially interfere in progress, but it comes down to focus, motivation and follow-through. There's no reason why a person can't carve out four hours to exercise each week. If they are in a very dysfunctional relationship where they aren't able to take care of themselves those issues may need professional attention and guidance, before it's reasonable to get oneself physically healthy. If this describes you, get professional help.

Interruptive relationships are ones where a combination of codependent and unsupportive dynamics come into play. If every time a person is headed to workout, eat healthy or take supplements someone close offers something that conflicts with your goals, you'll need to pay particular attention to prevent being distracted.

Self-development prerequisites:

There's a phenomena, in America, that has (in my opinion) seems to have increased over the last couple decades, since started working out and doing personal training where people seem to be missing fundamental stages of personal development, which inhibits their ability to reach their goals. It's not uncommon at all for personal trainers to receive requests or training from people who can't afford their fees.

Often being unhealthy out of shape, overweight, undernourished and so on are symptoms of poverty mindset, lack of self-worth, low self-esteem, unhealthy relationships and so on. Ironically, all those things seem to improve when people simply do resistance-training, cardio and nutrition. So, to me, this often begs the question, *"What's in between having the time, energy, resources and motivation to do a resistance-training, cardio and nutrition knowing all those life condition areas will likely improve, yet insist they can't do the program because they don't have the time, energy or resources?"* Do you hear the dichotomy, there?

For me, learning to exercise properly (my main motivation to get personal training) represented breaking the pattern/family dynamics of poverty & dysfunction. I felt that if I could learn to exercise, I would look and feel better, have a better life and grow away from the environment I had grown up in....live a more positive life, be around people who were more healthy and ultimately teach others what I had learned.

There's some presuppositions in there that life would improve, I had stuff to look forward to and my future would be brighter, in some way...although I didn't know that for sure...I was assuming it to be true and took action (time, energy and money) to find out. Truthfully, I got way more out of it than I expected. I had no idea how I felt about myself would improve so much. I think this qualifies as 'faith'. Faith that things would improve as a result of learning to exercise properly and the only evidence I had was that people I saw who worked out seemed happier and healthier than those who don't.

With that in mind, trainers get the people who want training but don't 'have' money to pay for training, gym membership (the budget money for coffee, alcohol, fast food and ice cream but can't afford supplements). Trainers get people who make their own schedule but don't set aside four hours a week for resistance and cardio (priorities). Trainers get people who won't eat enough food before their workouts to get through an hour of exercise (self-worth and discipline).

The point being that its common that the underlying symptoms and emotional strategies are the reason why they are in poverty, unfit, overweight and malnourished...essentially all symptoms of not managing their own life nor prioritizing themselves in their own life...effectively in reaction mode to what pops up in life instead of proactively creating the situations that support what they want their life to be about. If a person isn't willing to look at their life, it can seem that life is happening to them, is working against them...is out of reach for them...the common factor being how each person perceives their life...the point of view they are utilizing...which yes, often relates to early peer influence and skill sets used at home while growing up.

It's very common for trainers to hear clients reveal that they thought they could pay the trainer and get the results they have seen other people 'get', thinking that 'having a trainer', 'paying for training' is what produces results. It comes as a surprise that having a trainer usually means the workouts will be even more intense than working out on their own. It's very common for clients to be surprised that results come not from the four hours of exercise per week, but in the how they spend the other 164 hours in the week, mainly lifestyle related to the three parts of nutrition. It's pretty common, industry-wide that we tell our clients, *"80% of the results they get or miss out on is the result of the quality and timing of whole-foods, functional-foods and certain kinds of dietary supplements at certain times,"* yet, they give excuses why it doesn't fit for them and then complain they aren't getting results they want, seemingly thinking they are the one exception to science and nature.

Nutrition being 80% of what you have to 'do' during the week...if you skip those three parts, you're skipping 80% of what produces results, making excuses and then complaining about the results they think they deserve. People who skip the three parts of nutrition tend to insist that they can't get results from nutrition and exercise, that the laws of nature don't apply to them...they're different than everyone else...they are the one exception to nature and science!

Often, if people perceive they have the option of doing something to reach a goal or not, they skip it...that's why I screen potential clients nowadays so much. I simply don't want to waste the time of a person who doesn't want to invest their time, energy and resources to reach the goals they say they want and I certainly don't want to take my attention off the people who are making the way to invest their time, energy and resources. People have just as much right to succeed as fail and I personally work with the people who do what it takes to succeed, without excuses or reasons why they can't follow through. I specialize in working with do'ers.

One of the best kept secrets in the fitness industry is that if you want to slow down a clients' success to prolong their dependence on a trainer, leave out the three parts of a complete nutrition program.

I get a lot of questions on motivation. I have an entire book that discusses motivation, but next is a few tips that can really make a difference.

Chapter Nineteen

Some Insight On Motivation:

"Until you can discern between food & nutrition, progress and full mental capacity are not likely...the brain is directly dependent on the quality, quantity, timing and consistency of nutrition-density you put in your body or withhold from your body...motivation is a function which is dependent on a properly fueled/nourished brain."

-Sov Valentine, September 2016.

Did you know that a recent article published in June 2016 in BMJ entitled *"Ultra-processed foods and added sugars in the US diet: evidence from a nationally representative cross-sectional study,"* showed that the average American gets 57.9 percent of their calories from ultra-processed foods...that's foods that have had the nutrition-density processed out and then sold to livestock yards to feed to the livestock to keep them healthy for market.

http://bmjopen.bmj.com/content/6/3/e009892.full

I have found that it is a very common occurrence that the more the brain needs the B.N.B.B.s the more the person asks/insists for evidence...but fails to act on the evidence provided: *"...tell me a good supplement that no one is making money from"*. In other words, asking for a supplement but then adding the qualifier at the end *("...that no one is making money from.")* which effectively disqualifies all supplements...the malnourished brain doesn't hear the dichotomy of the question itself posed.

One of the most asked questions personal trainer get is, *"How do I get motivated...stay motivated?"*

When I first heard this, I had to really think back through my own life and record of reaching goals. I really couldn't figure out what that kind of questions means. I thought back to my own fitness successes...what preceded them? What preceded educational accomplishments? What about when I got a job I really wanted? Vacations goals and so on. Having come from an environment where the odds were against me and where people talked a lot about the reality they would rather have had but didn't do anything to get what they insisted they wanted, I went outside my immediate peer group to learn the behaviors of accomplishment (hint, hint).

It really never occurred to me that I was motivated, I simply do the steps to reach the goal and don't stop, instead of wishing or hoping something would magically happen or instead of trying to get someone to do my exercise and nutrition for me. I never question the steps to accomplishment, but rather do the steps and if they happen to not produce the kind of results I want, change them until they do (different than altering a plan to make it more comfortable or convenient or lowering the quality of the goal as the achievement date approaches). I assume the direction I'm given works until I notice that the actions (done properly and consistently) aren't producing results, in the suggested timeline.

The answer most people don't want to hear is that motivation is an inside job...it comes from and is cultivated within...it's not anything anyone can do 'to you' from the outside or 'make you' become. Even though, there's a percent of the population that believes life happens *to* them. When they see others reaching their goals they think it has to do with luck rather than hard work. People will think the same thing about you as you reach your goals...the work itself to reach goals is usually lonely.

I have seen patterns where a person believes someone should 'give' them energy and motivation to do what they want. This is common in unhealthy relationships, where the children were taking better care of the parents than the parents were of the children...the children develop a belief that any energy they get should be used to give to their parents...so inherent in that is that someone else will provide them with energy for motivation...an unnatural flow of energy.

Vicarious learning:

There's a common saying among business professionals and entrepreneurs that each person's income and success level will be the average of the five people they associate with the most. Although I haven't seen the scientific 'proof' of this being consistently true, I have seen and experienced what I believe the evidence that it's true. The major underlying theme that is outside conscious awareness is that whatever level of success a person is having in the major areas of life (relationships, career, income, health & fitness, recreation, etc.) is the next level of potential success.

In my professional opinion, after decades of this, the most significant factor is one's ability to become and stay motivated toward each goal is first and foremost the belief that they can achieve what they want to achieve (with the right amount of correct work). When one believes they can and they commit to putting in the work, many other forces come into play to make the thing happen. So, a single, great factor in going to the next level of anything is being able to see/visualize that it can be done. This begins by watching/studying/observing others do what it is you want to do. So, in this respect you can see that whom you're around has a direct influence on who you'll become. That is NOT to say you dump or give up on your current friends, family and associations...it implies that you'll 'add in' new/greater variety of associations (hopefully people who you aspire to have qualities similar to). In this respect, it's very common to hear Olympic medal winners talk about their obsession with their athletic role models, having their picture taken with their role models, essentially becoming fans and simultaneously imagining themselves living the reality of being on the winner's podium, until one day they too are on the podium.

I believe that every person we come into contact with can teach us a lesson regardless of their age or association to our current goals or interests...you just have to be open to receiving gifts from unexpected places. Sometimes these gifts come across as slips-of-the tongue, unconscious communication, answers to questions, demonstrations of courage and so on. All of which may come from a person who has no knowledge of your goals, aspirations, strengths, weaknesses, history, etc. In other words, talking to a person with an unrelated career, for example, if you have sincere interest in the person they may tell you something they think is about their truck driving experience, but directly answers a burning questions you have about yourself in relation to weight loss, strength, endurance and yes, recovery from injury...meaning, part of what keeps a person cut off from their own motivation, is being overly self-absorbed (behaving as if you'll solve the problem with the same state of mind that created the problem).

In this sense, it simply means find the people who have/are what you want to have/become and ask them to let you watch them doing the actions they do to get where they are. By simply being 'around' people that have what you want for your own life, the influence will be profound. This goes for recovering from chronic injuries as well. If it were me and I had in injury that was nagging and chronic, I'd find athletes who had successfully recovered from their injury and come back stronger and copy their daily routine...much of what they 'do' will be outside your awareness. The point being that you'll inadvertently/unconsciously learn the success habits of the person who overcame a weakness.

The people who don't get over their weaknesses are the ones who want to control 'how' they overcome their weakness, e.g. either they are trying to solve the problem with the same mindset and emotional state that created the problem (circular insanity) or they are so attached to 'how' the problem is solved that they literally block the solution...yes, I am saying that often, when people are having 'motivation' issues or trouble healing from an injury the problem has to do with control (or the illusion of control for the sake of perceived safety and security) more than a problem that doesn't have a solution or can't be solved...in other words, the issue is related more to emotionally attempting to stay the same, stop time and/or fear of moving toward/stepping into the reality of what they insist they want.

When I watch Olympic-level athletes, the successful ones have set aside emotional doubt, fear, insecurity, and yes even control. Once you've done the work you have to trust that the work you have done is enough and even in succeeding you're going to be ok. At a certain point, whether we're talking Olympics or permanent weight loss you have to let go of the old and make room, for the new with faith you'll be ok.

Chronic, recurrent injuries are more often related to stuck emotional states than physical limitations. In other words, if someone has made it through elementary, high school, collegiate and finally up to the ranks of professional and Olympic-levels any interference is directly related to stuck emotional-states that are just outside the athlete's conscious awareness. Metaphorically, there is a direct correlation, e.g. a person who unconsciously values being right all the time (control issue) might have a 'right' hamstring, glute, hip or shoulder problem that 'seems to have a mind of its own'. In this example, the tightness or muscular imbalance seems physical but if they have reached the upper echelon of their specialty it would be contrary to think one area of the body wouldn't be up to the challenge...it's emotional.

Where it can get a bit tricky in identifying the real problem is if, say for example, the person says they value going to the Olympics above all else, but in reality, they value having control more so. In this case, valuing control will show up as tightness in one area or muscle group of the body and most likely in the area that they use for their particular sport or activity the most...almost as if the body is saying, *"If you want to win, you have to let go of control,"* (the body knows what has to be done for it to perform its best even when the ego disagrees).

Delayed gratification:

I think one of the most common personality traits among people who are successful in fitness and athletics is delaying gratification. If you watched the daily actions of successful people versus those who claim to lack motivation or want someone else to motivate them from the outside, you would see the successful people doing exercise and nutrition strategies, which will have cumulative, long-term payoffs even if it means not having as much moment to moment gratification. The people who claim to lack motivation are more focused on doing behaviors that give them smaller payoffs of gratification, from moment-to-moment. Generally, the short-term payoffs tend to have de-motivating affects, on the mind and physiology, which interfere with doing the actions that provide long-term, yet big payoffs.

Inspiration vs motivation:

Ultimately, you have to cultivate your desire to succeed.

Inspiration comes from outside us. We hear a speech, a speaker, watch a movie, read a story, see someone being successful at something we want...something sparks us to *want* something...often seeing another person being, having, experiencing or doing a thing we want for ourselves. Sometimes the spark itself is a summary of all our life experiences...in other words, based on all we've experienced or wish we had experienced we begin imagining on something that will move us toward something (proactive-action) or get us away from something (reactive-action)...something that makes up for another thing...e.g. growing up in poverty vs being independently wealthy. Another example would be becoming lean, fit, strong and healthy having grown up in an unhealthy environment or an environment which promotes poor health, even if its subtle.

Proactive-action tends to be sustainable, but requires focus to keep yourself on track, since you keep fueling your own emotional drivers beyond the first action to start the course to achieve what you want through small, cumulative action and accomplishment. Proactive-action requires holding yourself accountable, even when no one is watching or holding you accountable...just doing it.

Reactive-action tends to be intermittent, since once the intense, but fleeting emotions that started to get us away from a thing wanes, so does the actions which would have gotten us truly away to a different level of being. Reactive-action serves as a coping mechanism to help a person deal with stress, in the moment, but lacks the integrity to follow through, once the emotions of the situation have been 'vented'.

In order to follow through, stick to the path and keep the emotional-fire burning. To reach a goal you have to go from inspiration (short-term outside influence) to motivation (long-term, internally driven self-discipline) to form a daily routine of the work required to reach the goal (habits) which turn into as a lifestyle which supports what you insisted you wanted to be, posses, experience or do (goal-achievement).

Some people are raised in an environment where reaching goals is inherent in the peer group...meaning its demonstrated and expected that you apply yourself and work toward what you say you want until you achieve it, so the payoff of the hard work is seen early on. Others may have the deck stacked against them, needing to go outside themselves to earn the knowledge of achievement, having no base of experience related to seeing the value of hard work, follow through & accomplishment.

Simplicity:

A common factor is achievement is keeping things simple:

■ Want the thing (decide what you want),

■ Start taking CORRECT action,

■ Initial results fuel motivation for improvement and efficiency (requires faith you'll succeed),

■ Noticing/measuring/keep track how well/if what you're doing is working to reach your goal on time,

■ Adjusting and refining to get more efficient (same results for less time, energy & money),

■ Get professional help if you don't know what to do next or have hit a plateau,

■ Retain whatever information you gain: (trainers & coaches know who is serious by who retains the information that has been passed onto them, and who applies what was taught),

■ Copying people who have already been successful (modeling) or getting professional help from a professional who can truly help you (mentoring),

■ Focus (doing your action while others are doing actions for their own goals),

■ Holding yourself accountable (don't give yourself permission to get off track),

■ Self-discipline (just do it and keep doing it) and

■ Consistency and refinement (keep going until you reach your goal).

Before I got a personal trainer (Tracy) I watched tons of episodes of cable TV fitness shows to learn how to exercise my abs, lying on the floor in the living room after early morning shifts on the dairy farm. Once I had gotten as far as I could from the TV shows I sought professional help! I got the help and did exactly what Tracy showed me to do, without trying to change it or make excuses.

Earn & learn:

When people say they want someone there to motivate them, it's like asking for free money...you have to earn it...not so much to 'get it' but to keep it. The value of a dollar is relative to how much energy was exerted to get the dollar and motivation is the same way...the more you put into the actions to get what results you've gotten, the more you want to keep the results and prevent having to start over...your lifestyle determines if you're building in more motivation to yourself or interfering/interrupting in your own motivation. You control your motivation.

Remember the cliche, *"You can lead a horse to water, but you can't make them drink?"* Motivation is the same way...it's really a misunderstanding in the use of the mind: If someone has to drag you along then you really don't want to earn what you say you want or you want other people to be responsible for your emotions!

And that can happen: some people don't know that how people achieve their goals is NOT by being drug along like a horse that isn't thirsty. Most of goal-achievement is personal responsibility. There's no individual on the planet who can do the work for another (otherwise they would do the work for themselves). And there's no person who can maintain a goal for you once achieved it (indicated by the fact that everyone s living their own life...it's called freedom!). If you want someone to continually motivate you, you're effectively asking others to use some of their life force to feed your life...that's neither balanced, healthy nor sustainable. The fastest way to burn out a trainer or training partner or family member for that matter is to constantly demand they carry you emotionally ("Motivate me").

And there's no magical amount of money that you could pay anyone to do the work for you, since no matter how much you would pay a person, they would be exchanging money for reaching their own goals...they might have a goal of having money, but there's a lot easier and more efficient ways to earn money than dragging a horse to get a drink when they could just give drinks to horses who are ready for the water!...or get a drink themselves.

Motivation is something you initiate based on what you want so bad you don't want to go on any longer, at least not working toward it.

Once you start the process, self-discipline comes into play. Without self-discipline, how do you expect to get anything out of life? There's no free rides that are worth it or sustainable in the long run. It's not uncommon for people to need to improve and develop their self-discipline as they go along and refine the process of moving themselves toward their goals. One of the most common motivators for people who had a challenging time getting going is the idea of losing what they have gained from their health and fitness habits...once you get it, you don't want to lose it, you want to get more of it!

If you lack self-discipline study self-discipline *as you're doing* the actions to meet your goals. Nothing replaces doing exercise and nutrition...nothing. So, start, get going and adjust course as you learn more. The person who wants others to do the work for them will also blame others for the results they didn't get from the work they didn't do!

One of the ways seasoned trainers check the emotional-stability and clarity of potential clients is by asking what they think their doctor or trainer will tell them they have to do to reach their goals. The answers that come next will clearly identify whether a person wants to get the benefits of exercise and nutrition and is prepared to get to work or if they are simply wanting someone else to fix them or provide the magic pill. These answers indicate the person's beliefs about work ethic, how reasonable they are, how rational they are and if their expectations are realistic as well as emotional clarity. People who haven't reached their goals and tell story after story of what hasn't worked are often chronic self-distracters...they do anything but what works.

Part of the way experienced trainers find out where a person is misleading themselves is in the initial consultation/interview. Chronic-distracters categorically obsess over outdated health information...for example, insisting they need to eliminate all fat from their diet, overtly focus on cutting calories or eliminating carbohydrates from their nutritional program, etc....by focusing on what is already proven to not work and hurt the health. The more one reduces calories, the more critical dietary supplements are...the less food you eat the more you have to get your nutrition from dietary supplements...where does the nutrition come from if you aren't eating it!? Whole-foods have to be the basis/foundation/cornerstone of the three parts of nutrition, but why would you leave it to chance? If your goals are that important why would you leave the thing that has to be in place to chance? You wouldn't. Think about it.

The chronic-distracter avoids accountability...unfortunately, the more malnourished a person, the less likely their brain will be able to take in and retain the very information they need. There reaches a point where a person is so accustomed to being malnourished they aren't likely to succeed. One of the hallmarks of a chronic-distracter client is that they don't do what their trainer says, but attempt to distract their trainer by referring other friends, co-workers and family to their trainer in attempt to distract from the fact that they aren't doing their part. It's common. Referrals are great, but a person who isn't doing their part generally refer more people who won't do their part!

"Cognitive, subpar-nutrition is when a person insists on skipping one or more of the three parts of nutrition (whole foods, functional-foods and certain kinds of dietary supplements at certain times) to the point where their brain doesn't mentally function well enough to comprehend to put nutrition in, thereby shifting behavioral function from a mental activity (choosing action based on healthy choice and cumulative health benefits) to an (emotional-based activity, where choices are based on emotional relief moment to moment), regardless of affects on health, in the long run, let alone stated health and fitness goals."

Sovereign Valentine, September 2016

In order to achieve goals, you've never achieved or go to the next level, you have to sort out the emotions related to the goals, clear up the inner-conflicts and move behavioral function from emotional-based activity to higher level, cognitive functioning (simply do what works) without contaminating it with contrary thoughts, ideas and inner dialogue.

Training partners:

It's not uncommon for the new fitness buff to think they need a training partner to motivate them to show up and workout out...again, a misunderstanding. No individual wants to show up for their own workout only to have to drag another person through their workouts too (boring and energy-sucking).

I can tell you from experience, that the best training partners are bringing just as much to the session as they are getting from the session. Each person will have their own strengths (physical, mental, emotional, spiritual) and they'll both have their own goals that their partner takes into account and helps them with from one set to another, rep by rep. A big part of having a great partnership in a training partner comes down to being 'present'. Being present meaning you and your partner are totally focused and there to help each other do things you can't do by yourselves.

I've seen the one-sided training partners who insist you spot them and help them get through their set, but when it's time to return the favor they're off talking to people in the gym, texting, talking on the phone, missing spots and so forth. Having a great training partners means consideration for the other person...not being focused simply on what you'll get from them. This should go without saying, but then this comes down to relationship dynamics and it's not uncommon either for one partner to convince their partner to be present during the workout...as if they have to train their training partner how to be a training partner!

You can just about tell within the first couple exercises if your partner is there to give as much as get simply by how much they're paying attention. Both people should bring energy to the training session...energy for themselves! If you have to motivate your partner, you don't have a partner you have a therapy client. Secondly, your partner should be there to help you bring out the best in yourself. If they don't eat right to fuel (ignoring nutrition), show up late, leave early and so on it's not a match and it won't be (mismatch of values).

Because fitness does require physical, mental and emotional energy, it's a common pattern that the people who want others to motivate them are either not cultivating their own energy (poor nutrition, unhealthy thoughts and mindset, sloppy lifestyle, lack of discipline, lack of time out in nature). In other words their lifestyle is using up energy but not returning or cultivating energy OR they're giving away energy to others whom are also 'takers' (a circle of people giving energy away too much in hopes some will be given back, based on the erroneous ideas that you're a better person for giving of the self which you haven't earned to give away) OR simply being so stagnant in their life that they haven't done the actions to overcome inertia (the resistance of any physical object to any change in its state of motion, including changes to its speed, direction or state of rest). In other words, you have to do it yourself. Start small. Be consistent. Increase the quality and quantity as you go.

Procrastination (opposite of motivation) is timeless. Ancient Greek philosophers like Aristotle and Socrates coined the term akrasia: the state of acting against your better judgment...It is when you do one thing even though you know you should do something else...loosely translated, you could say that akrasia is procrastination or a lack of self-control...it's what prevents you from following through on what you set out to do.

On the other hand, they also coined enkrateia: *"...to be in power over yourself"*.

"Happiness depends upon ourselves." –Aristotle

You can do it!

Ask me for help.

"Until one is committed, there is hesitancy, the chance to draw back. Concerning all acts of initiative (and creation), there is one elementary truth that ignorance of which kills countless ideas and splendid plans: that the moment one definitely commits oneself, then Providence moves too. All sorts of things occur to help one that would never otherwise have occurred. A whole stream of events issues from the decision, raising in one's favor all manner of unforeseen incidents and meetings and material assistance, which no man could have dreamed would have come his way. Whatever you can do, or dream you can do, begin it. Boldness has genius, power, and magic in it. Begin it now."

Johann Wolfgang von Goethe
1749-1832

Pre-training Questionnaire:

Have you had professional nutrition training before? ___Yes ___No

Are you coachable and open to whole-foods nutrition suggestions?
___Yes ___No
Would you follow through on my suggestions?   ___Yes ___No

Did you know that your fitness/fat-loss success or lack thereof is about 80%, based on the how well you apply the three parts of nutrition, during/from the first month, of your program?
___Yes ___No
Have you had professional B.N.B.B.s training?
___Yes ___No

Are you coachable and open to suggestions about which B.N.B.B.s to take, for optimal results? (versus picking a program apart).
___Yes ___No

Currently participating in a structured, resistance-training?
___Yes ___No
If so, frequency/duration of sessions ?_________________________.

Have you had professional personal training before? ___Yes ___No

Have you had fat-burning cardio-respiratory training before?
___Yes ___No

Is it realistic for you to prioritize 3-4 hours [each week] to exercise?
___Yes ___No

What is your current bodyfat percentage?_________________________.

How much fat do you want to lose?_________________________.

What has been your biggest challenge(s), in regard to fat-loss?

____.

Are you committed to applying yourself to resistance-training, cardiovascular-training, and the 3 parts of nutrition: (1) Whole-foods, 2) Functional-foods, & 3) The B.N.B.B.s *for at least one year?* (versus a person who starts stuff, but doesn't follow through).

___Yes ___No

With a standard of 12-20 pounds per month, how long could it take you to lose amount of fat, you intend to lose_______________________________.
How many different weight loss programs have you tried, before?

____.

I look for people who have tried a few things that didn't work and who are looking for something that definitely works. Are you the type of person who wants a structured program that tells you exactly what to do throughout the day, so nothing is left to chance?

___Yes ___No

Are you willing to get your B.N.B.B.s squared away, from the beginning of your program?

___Yes ___No

Although you will likely begin to see and feel positive improvements right away, permanent fat-loss requires a lifestyle change. Are you willing to become more fit by committing to a program that definitely works, for at least one year? (versus a short-term quick fix).

___Yes ___No

How long have you been wanting to lose weight?__________________.

Imagine you have lost all the fat you ever wanted to, have more energy and look better than ever and all that is taken care of. In what way(s) would your life improve, as a result?

____

*You may find it helpful to remove these pages, scan them and email them to me to assist with your complimentary consultation.

Afterword

How I like to work is to do an initial consultation/interview, with people who want my help. During this time, I screen people for particular characteristics, which indicate if this is a good program match for them or not, explain my fees, what is expected and so forth. I am a fairly tough trainer, since clients expect a lot for their money and in turn I expect accountability, so you get your money's worth...but these are some of the reasons my clients get such good results.

How I know a person is serious and ready to be a client and how I take you seriously is when you get your whole-foods, functional-foods and B.N.B.B.s lined up for at least weeks in advance. You have to have your supplies ready in advance and replenish them before you run out. This is sometimes considered a serious program, since there's no days that go by that you aren't sticking to the plan. You're either in/on it or you're not...there's no modified program.

Once I'm convinced you're serious and a good candidate, and you've purchased a copy of this book I'll email the eight-week journal and shopping list to help make sure you have everything you need to succeed and get the most from each of your eight-week cycles.

Contact me via email and we'll set up a preliminary phone appointment from there. If you choose to hire me as your trainer to get going on this program, I'll be in consistent contact with you, to make sure you're on track and answer your questions, offer morale support and help you succeed on your program.

One of the most commonly asked question by my clients, after a few weeks on this program is, *"Why are my hair, skin and nails looking so much better than they ever have before?"*

I look forward to working with you.

As a licensed health care provider, author, speaker and fitness professional I know from my own experiences what it feels like to want to improve my health, do what I think is right and still not get the kind of results I expected. I am sure you have your own goals and are looking forward to achieving them. I believe you are capable of living the life of your dreams in your healthy, ideal-self body and you will achieve your dreams.

I want you to contact me today and tell me about all the positive benefits you have experienced, as a result of this information!

In my experience, the greatest potential problem is in not educating yourself about it, but in simply doing it.

I cannot wait to hear from you. I especially cannot wait to share your success story with others.

Appendix

For your complimentary consultation, contact the author at the email below or through Facebook Messenger at Sov Valentine:

e-mail:

sovereignmv@gmail.com

My website:

http://sovereign-valentine.mykajabi.com

Sovereign Valentine
CFT, CET, Yft, SSC, SPN, SSF, Cft, GFI, SFI, EMR, CERT, CMCht, Reiki Master

Reasons or Results! Training Systems© 2018

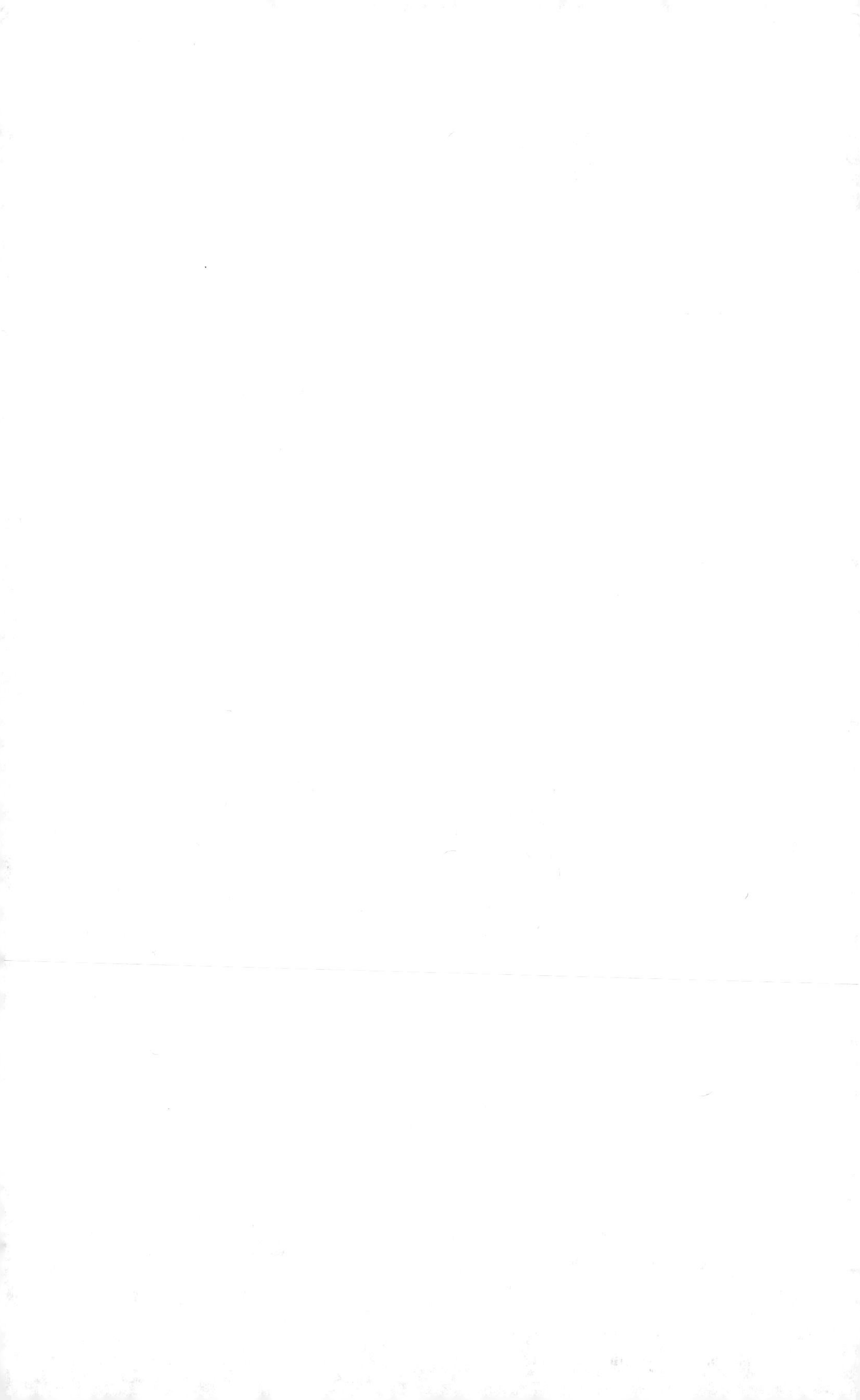